THE TAO OF
Nutrition

NEW AND EXPANDED EDITION

MAOSHING NI, Ph.D., C.A.
With CATHY McNEASE, B.S., M.H.

Foreword by HUA-CHING NI

Published by:
SevenStar Communications Group, Inc.
13315 W. Washington Boulevard Suite 200
Los Angeles, CA 90066
WWW.SevenStarCom.com

The paper used in this publication meets the minimum requirements of the American National Standard for Information Sciences Permanence of Paper for Printed Library Materials, ANSI 239.48-1984.

First Printing January 1987
Second Printing February 1989
Third Printing June 1991
Fourth Printing June 1993
Fifth Printing March 1996
Sixth Printing February 1998
Seventh Printing June 2000
Eighth Printing December 2004

Library of Congress Cataloging-in-Publication Data
Ni, Maoshing.
        The Tao of nutrition / by Maoshing Ni, with Cathy McNease. –
rev. ed.
        p.   cm.
        Includes bibliographical references and index.
        ISBN 0-937064-66-1 : $14.95
        1.   Nutrition. 2. Health--Religious aspects--Taoism. 3. Diet therapy.
I. McNease, Cathy. II. Title.   93-7783
RA784.N5 1987b   CIP
613.2—dc20

DEDICATION
Eat not for the pleasure thou mayest find therein. Eat to increase thy strength. Eat to preserve the life thou has received from heaven. Confucius

ACKNOWLEDGEMENT
I would like to express my deepest gratitude to my father who has endowed me with this great tradition and knowledge so that I may be able to share them with everyone. A special appreciation to Cathy McNease who untiringly transcribed all my lectures into readable form and helped to arrange and edit the text into this final version. Without her help, this book would not have become available. Thanks to Charlie Blythe for his many generous hours of computer work to produce this new revision.

We would also like to thank all of our students, patients and friends for their valuable suggestions and feedback with the remedies in this book. To everyone who continues to support and promote natural medicine in this world, we are most grateful to all of you.

DISCLAIMER
This book is intended to present to the reader the energetic and the healing aspects of foods. It is the authors' desire to help those who are open minded about natural alternatives to healing. However, the remedies offered within, are to the authors' best knowledge and experience and are to be used by readers at their own discretion. If you wish to try the therapeutic approaches outlined in this book for serious conditions, we advise you to find a doctor of Oriental Medicine that is familiar with the field of Chinese Nutrition who can supervise you in your treatment program.

ABOUT THE AUTHORS

Maoshing Ni, born into a family of medical traditions as the thirty-eighth generation of traditional Chinese healers, began his training early in life. He studied intensively with his father, a Taoist Master and a Master healer, and many other teachers in the subjects of Chinese Medicine, martial arts, Tai Chi Chuan, Taoism and other related arts in China. He attended schools in China and the United States and received advanced degrees and license as an acupuncturist. He is the co-founder and vice president of Yo San University of Traditional Chinese Medicine, and is presently in private practice in Santa Monica.

Cathy McNease is an herbalist and writer living in California with her husband. Together they own a Chinese herb business and teach classes in herbalism, Chinese Nutrition and related subjects. Cathy is on the faculty of two acupuncture colleges, a member of the American Herbalists Guild, and co-author of *101 Vegetarian Delights*. She received degrees with honors from Western Michigan University and Emerson College of Herbology, and has studied under some of the most notable herbalists in this country. Much of her interest in nutrition and herbs began twenty years ago when she became a vegetarian. As a student of the Taoist tradition and the Ni family, she continues to further her training in the Chinese healing arts.

TABLE OF CONTENTS

LIST OF RECIPES

FOREWORD

The knowledge of nutrition in China has roots that go back at least 6,000 years and is based on the principles of balance and harmony, as well as direct knowledge of the nature of individual foods. This knowledge was first gathered by spiritually achieved men and women who, by their own experiences, learned not only what properties specific foods contained, but also how to utilize them for the purposes of nutrition and longevity. Anyone who learns and uses this ancient, time-tested knowledge will find their health and longevity greatly enhanced.

Fu Shi, one of the great sages of ancient China, discovered eight categories of universal energy, which later came to be known as the *Ba Gua* or *Eight Trigrams*; this is a further division of the two main categories of natural energy known as Yin and Yang. The universe itself is an integration of these two interacting, mutually assisting and also somewhat opposing forces which are often expressed by the *Tai Chi* symbol illustrated on the front cover of this book.

The deepest reality of universal life is the inner meaning of Yin and Yang, and, like Yin and Yang, the nature of the universe also tends to be both harmonious and balanced. Even events which could be conceptually classified as negative or conflicting, are only stages in the accomplishment of further harmonization. This is the truth expressed in the *Tai Chi* diagram.

Harmony and balance, therefore, the principles of universal existence, became the foundation of cultural development in ancient China and were widely applied in public and private life as well as in spiritual practice. Many generations later, whatever expressed these natural universal qualities of balance, harmony and symmetry came to be known as *Taoism: Tao* being the way or path of universal harmony through integration.

Shen Nung, another wise leader who lived some time after Fu Shi, used these principles to develop herbal medicine and essential nutrition. After him came the Yellow Emperor, one of the greatest leaders in human history, who has come to be considered the *founder* of Taoism. He further developed the contributions of the early sages, utilizing them in political as well as general life, especially in the realms of medicine and nutrition, and benefiting his hundred-year reign greatly by the guidance of this special knowledge.

Fu Shi, Shen Nung and the Yellow Emperor are great symbols of natural culture. Another symbolic figure of longevity is popular even now in Chinese culture. He is called Pung Tzu and is considered the founder of the art of Chinese cooking and nutrition. Pung Tzu learned all the arts of long life, including *Do-In*, energy conducting exercises, and *Fang Zhong*, the art and discipline of sexual practices. Legend has it that Pung Tzu lived to be 800 years old and was still active in the reign of the Emperor Jou, around 1123 B.C.

As the spiritual descendants of these men of spiritual development and dedication to human development, we can still benefit today from their great achievements and contributions, as many have done before us. Through the traditional Chinese healing arts and herbal medicine, I myself have offered much useful knowledge and help to many people around the world. Although I taught a class on diet and nutrition several years ago, there was still a secret wish in my mind to do more in this area. Because of my busy schedule, I have not had time to do so, but fortunately my son, Maoshing, had the same interest. Thus, he has brought this book into your hands to fill the gap in my own work. It can be an important and useful tool in your life that will serve your health and spiritual development. With its support, I wish that each of you may become stronger every day.

Thank you,

Ni, Hua-Ching
January 1987
Los Angeles, CA.

PREFACE

In a rapidly changing society such as ours, people have lost their instinctive nature in the ways of eating. People have a poor concept of what makes up a good diet. They thrive and rely on their taste buds and visual sensations for sustenance. In most cases, they have not learned to eat to live, but rather live to eat. Even more sadly, caught in the daily rat race of their surroundings, many people take priority for work, pleasure, and sex over what they eat. Also, at the same time mind boggling numbers of different fads and controversial dietary regimes add even more confusion to the already uncertain dietary habits of today's people. All of these show in the deterioration of the quality of people's lives in modern society.

The Tao of Nutrition presents the wisdom of the ancient Chinese. Ancient people were much more aware of the environment and how their bodies reacted to their surroundings. They lived by the principle of being in harmony with Nature and emphasized balance in every aspect of life, especially diet, the Yin and Yang of foods and of the body. Their knowledge and experiences were passed down through generations for many centuries, and further refined and systematized into what we today call Chinese Nutrition.

The system of Chinese Nutrition is a healing system of its own. Not only is it a healing system, but also a disease prevention system. The advantage of Chinese Nutrition lies in its flexibility in adapting to every individual's needs, and treating the whole person instead of the disease.

Chinese Nutrition differs from modern Western nutrition in that it does not rely on analyzing the chemical constituents of each food; rather, it determines the properties or energies of each food and combination, taking into consideration season, method of preparation, and geographical

location, and utilizes the information according to the
natural principles of life and balance.

It is hoped that the readers of this book will gain insight
and understanding into their bodies, their surroundings, and
their diet. So here it is, the essence of the art and science of
Chinese Nutrition. With this book in your hands you can be
the master of your own body. Start now to better yourself
and other people to achieve and maintain health, vitality,
and longevity.

HOW TO USE THIS BOOK

This book contains three major sections: Section 1 deals with theories and philosophies of Chinese Nutrition; Section 2 describes over 130 common foods in detail (their energetic properties, their therapeutic actions, and individual remedies); and Section 3 is a remedial section which gives recommendations for various medical conditions.

It is strongly recommended that readers familiarize themselves thoroughly with Section 1 in order to understand the basic philosophies of Chinese Nutrition. With that understanding, one is able to more efficiently utilize the specific knowledge given in Sections 2 and 3.

Another way readers may find this book useful is to utilize it according to what condition may apply to them. So they may choose to look up a specific condition in Section 3 and follow the recommendations given there. Or check the index for all listings of the condition.

For example, if you look up *Headache* in Section 3, you will find the following therapeutic remedies to choose from: FOR HEADACHES DUE TO COMMON COLD OR FLU:

1. Make tea from ginger and green onions, boiling for 5 minutes; drink and try to sweat.

2. Steam aching portion of head over mint and cinnamon tea that is cooking, then dry head afterwards, avoiding catching a draft.

3. Make tea from chrysanthemum flowers and cassia seeds and drink.

4. Make buckwheat meal into a paste and apply to painful area until it sweats.

5. Drink green tea.

2

6. Make rice porridge and add garlic and green onions. Eat while hot, then get under covers and sweat.

FOR HEADACHES DUE TO HIGH BLOOD PRESSURE, MENSTRUAL CYCLES, EMOTIONAL STRESS OR TENSION, OR MIGRAINES:

1. Make carrot juice. If headache is on left side, squirt carrot juice into left nostril; if on right side, squirt into right nostril; if both sides are painful, squirt into both nostrils.

2. Take lemon juice and 1/2 T. baking soda mixed in a glass of water and drink.

3. Make tea of Chinese prunes, mint, and green tea.

4. Make tea of oyster shells and chrysanthemum flowers, slowly boiling the shells for 1 1/2 hours, then adding the flowers for the last 30 minutes.

5. Mash peach kernels and walnuts, mix with rice wine and lightly roast it; take 2 T. 3 times daily.

6. Rinse head with warm water, gradually increasing the temperature to hot.

After studying the entire book, one will gain an insight into maintaining balance and harmony with one's body and environment and ultimately achieve health, happiness and longevity.

SECTION

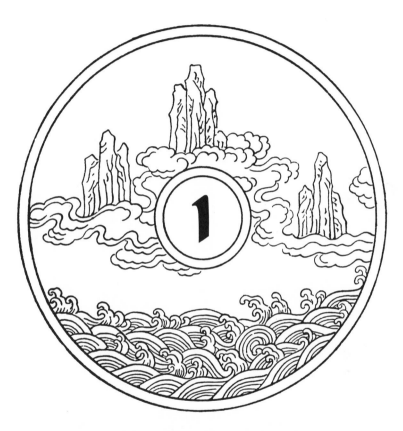

Introduction

Energetic Properties

Chinese Nutrition applies the traditional healing properties of foods to correct disharmonies within the body. Over the course of several millennia, countless experiences were gathered using food for prevention and healing of disease. This treasure was passed along as an important healing art, within the body of information known as Traditional Chinese Medicine.

Chinese Nutrition differs from Western nutrition in that it does not talk about the biochemical nature of food. Rather, Chinese Nutrition deals on an energetic level to which **balance is the key.** Foods are selected according to their energetic qualities such as warming, cooling, drying, or lubricating. Thus, Chinese Nutrition would seek to warm the coldness, cool the heat, dry the dampness, lubricate the dryness and so forth.

By carefully studying the individual's imbalances, one would choose the appropriate foods to bring about a balanced state of health. For example, for an excessive individual who is exhibiting conditions of heat in the body, cooling foods would be appropriate. For a deficient individual who tends toward coldness, warming foods would be chosen. In this way health is achieved.

Foods all have specific qualities inherent within, determined by the effect the food has on the body. Then the method of preparation either enhances or neutralizes the foods. Generally speaking, warming foods raise metabolism and cooling foods lower metabolism. Balance in the diet is essential for good health.

Yin and Yang

It is a universal law that everything is constantly changing, except for the fundamental governing laws of life. This principle applies to the universe surrounding us as well as the inner universe of our bodies. The ancient Chinese developed ways of looking at these changes to better understand them. One such theory is that everything in the universe consists of two opposite yet complementary aspects. This is called the *Theory of Yin and Yang*. Yin and Yang exist relative to one another and are also in a state of change at any given time; they are not static conditions. Day and night are a good example of this. When Yin and Yang are out of balance diseases or disharmonies occur.

Within the body, Yin and Yang are often referred to as the body's water and fire. These descriptions are very useful in determining the relative nature of both the individual and the energies of foods. The application of Chinese Nutrition necessitates determining the body type of the individual. He or she may be the *cold type*, considered of a Yin nature, the *hot type*, considered Yang, or, commonly a mixture. Some significant questions to determine this may be as follows, with the Yang tendencies listed first: male or female? feel hot or cold? drawn to cold or hot foods? thirst or no thirst? constipated or loose stools? dark or pale urine? red face or tongue or pale?

We are all a mixture of Yin and Yang, although we may be predominantly one or the other. Thus, Yang persons need relatively more Yin (cooling) foods and Yin types need relatively more Yang (warming) foods. Chinese Nutrition categorizes foods according to the observed reactions within the body. Easily observable changes occur according to the warming or cooling nature of a food. Foods are categorized as Hot, Warm, Neutral, Cool and Cold. (*Refer to Chart 1: Energetic Properties of Foods*)

Typical symptoms of the *hot type* or Yang type person could include the following: red complexion, easy to sweat, always hot, dominating, aggressive or outgoing personality, coarseness, loud voice, dry mouth, thirst, affinity to cold liquids, ferocious appetite, constipation, foul breath, scanty and dark urine, sometimes dry cough with thick yellow sputum, easily angered, very emotional, irritability, insomnia, and in women, early and heavy menstruation with bright red blood.

Typical symptoms of the *cold type* or Yin type could include the following: paleness, coldness, disdains cold liquids, likes warm liquids, low energy, loose stools, sleeps a lot, feeble and weak voice, introverted personality, white and copious sputum, lack of appetite, copious and clear urine, dizziness, and edema.

To bring about balance and counteract the symptoms, *hot type* persons would use primarily cooling foods such as wheat, mung beans, watermelon, fresh fruit juices, and many of the vegetables. *Cold type* persons would achieve balance by regularly including the warming foods in their diet, such as garlic, ginger, onions, black beans, lamb and chicken. Accordingly, *hot types* would avoid hot, spicy foods, while *cold types* would avoid cold, raw foods.

Yin and Yang also apply to the organs of our bodies. Those which are considered solid, or with substance, are considered Yin. These include Heart, Spleen, Liver, Lungs, Kidneys. Those which are considered hollow, active in transportation, are considered Yang. These include Large and Small Intestines, Gall Bladder, Stomach, and Urinary Bladder. Further descriptions of each organ and their energetic components will follow. (*Refer to Chart 2*)

Your Body Is The Greatest Healer

Americans are a perfect example of an overfed and undernourished country. We are constantly bombarded by information on nutrition from food companies, current faddists, and diet cultists, yet the picture is very incomplete.

According to the Chinese point of view, the body is looked at as a whole, working together in harmony. Just as every little screw and bolt on a machine has an important purpose, if one part is broken the whole suffers. Our body is a very intricate machine that works together as a whole.

Western medicine tends to focus on only the diseased part of the body. Then it tries to attack and kill the diseased cells, not taking into account why those cells are diseased to begin with. It is not just because the cells are exposed to viruses and bacteria. We are constantly exposed to these; our mouth is full of bacteria. Yet why is it that some people break down and get sick and others do not, when both are exposed to the same pathogens?

Our body is equipped with a healing mechanism that is greater than any invention. It is so unique that it has this system that can repair the body's disharmonies, given the right chance to do so. Through inappropriate lifestyle, diet, thoughts, and actions, we abuse the workings of this delicate system. Always keep in mind that the body's own healing system is very powerful. Suppressing a headache with aspirin does not take away the underlying cause. The headache is a warning of some disharmony. Thus, we should work on the underlying cause and use natural healing methods to enhance the immune system so the body can heal itself.

We should help the body to heal, not interfere with it. Often our surroundings do not give us the proper chance to heal ourselves, beginning with the bombardment of chemicals into our soil, food, water, and life, in general. These chemicals can accumulate in the liver and become very toxic.

Significant chemical pollution occurs in meats. Meat animals are routinely injected with steroids (Bovine Growth Hormones) to fatten them quickly and produce more milk. Antibiotics, including penicillin and sulfa, are used to control rampant diseases. These drug residues remain in the meat and milk and can cause a lot of problems to the consumer. The hormones can cause men to become more feminine and have problems with impotency and sterility, and women to experience premature aging and general disharmonies in their endocrine systems and menstrual cycles.

Traditional Chinese View of the Body

According to Traditional Chinese Medicine (TCM), the human being is an intricate whole, made up of these essential components: Chi (vital energy), blood, body fluids, Jing, and Shen (spirit). If any one of these components is missing, you cannot have life.

Chi comes in many forms with many different actions. In general, Chi is like life force. The body is a network of pathways filled with Chi called meridians. In a healthy person this Chi or energy flows evenly along these channels. When the energy becomes blocked, disease results. Acupuncture can be of great value to facilitate the flow of energy through these pathways. Chi (the Yang component) is closely related to blood (the Yin component). Blood supplies the nutritive aspect in the body and nourishes Chi. Movement of blood is dependent upon the Chi.

Body fluids are of two types: Jin are the thin, refined fluids such as sweat, tears, and tissue fluids and Ye are the thick, lubricating fluids such as spinal fluid and synovial (joint) fluids.

Jing is the *essence of life* found in the eggs, sperms, bone marrow, and the brain (*the sea of marrow*) and is stored in the Kidneys. At the time of conception, the fetus absorbs this vital essence from the egg and the sperm. All of our chromosomes at that time give us our Jing. Thus, we are born with a certain amount. Then throughout our lives we use up our Jing until we die. The fast-paced American lifestyle uses up Jing at a very rapid rate. For this reason women here have tremendous problems with menstruation, go through an earlier menopause and cannot safely bear children for as many years as in more natural cultures.

Spiritual cultivation is very important for the proper development and preservation of our Jing, which is stored in the Kidney. The Shen or spirit gives us intuition, instincts, and the ability to comprehend. Shen is housed in the Heart.

Organs of the Body

TCM views the body organs as couples consisting of a Yin organ and a Yang organ. Each pair also has energetic correlations that we may not necessarily associate with the physical organ. For example, the Kidneys in Chinese medicine would also include functions of the reproductive organs. Each pair of organs is associated with one of five energies called the Five Elements: Wood, Fire, Earth, Metal, and Water. The quality of the element is reflected in its organ pair.

The pair related to the Wood element is the Liver and Gall Bladder. The Liver houses the soul, controls tendons, is responsible for keeping the energy flowing (thus, when the energy is obstructed, look to the Liver), stores blood, and manifests externally in the eyes. Anger (as well as frustration and depression) relates to the Liver. The Gall Bladder stores and excretes bile, protects the nervous system from overreaction, and helps to normalize a person emotionally. Gall Bladder weakness may manifest as difficulty making decisions.

Corresponding to Fire are the Heart and Small Intestines. The Heart houses the Shen, governs blood, externally manifests in the tongue, has taste as its sensory function, and joy (mania) as its related emotion. The Small Intestines absorb fluids and as one of the hollow organs are responsible for the transporting of excretions.

Also related to the Fire element are the Triple Heater (Sanjiao) and the Pericardium which are functions rather than organs. The Triple Heater is responsible for communication between the three cavities in the trunk and helps with fluid metabolism in the body. The Pericardium surrounds and protects the Heart.

Corresponding to the element of Earth is the pair, Spleen and Stomach. The Spleen transforms and transports food into usable food essence (the waste is transported to the intestines), produces blood, opens to the mouth, controls muscles, and is responsible for keeping the blood in the vessels (thus, bruising easily is a sign of weak Spleen function). The related emotion is worry (excessive thinking). Reference made to the Spleen in the Chinese system also includes functions of the pancreas. The Stomach breaks down and *ripens* the food and then, transports it downward.

The pair corresponding to the Metal element is the Lungs and Large Intestines. The main functions of the Lungs are breathing, regulating water metabolism, and to descend and disperse the Chi throughout the body; Lungs open out to the nose, and control the skin, pores, and skin hair. Sadness is the related emotion. The Large Intestines excrete wastes from the body and absorb water.

Related to the Water element are the Kidneys and Urinary Bladder. The Kidneys store Jing, are responsible for growth, development, and reproduction, produce marrow, form brain and spinal cord, control bones, open to the ears, and balance body fluid metabolism. The related emotion is fear. The Urinary Bladder stores and excretes urine. (*Refer to Chart 2: Five Elements Correspondences*)

Five Elements

A useful theory in the Chinese view of the universe is the Five Elements Theory or the Five Energy Transformations. *(Refer to Chart 3)* This gives us a helpful framework to understand the ever-changing world, the inner relationships of change, and the interconnectedness of all things. The five elements, Wood, Fire, Earth, Metal, and Water, connect in that sequence for what is called the *creation cycle.* This cycle occurs in nature as well as within our bodies. In nature, rub two pieces of wood together and create fire; fire burns to ash and becomes earth; from earth we dig up metal; melt the metal to liquid and make water; put a seed into the water and it germinates a tree and creates wood. It is a circular and repetitive cycle.

In the *creation cycle* the creator element is the mother who gives birth to the son element. Thus, if the son is weak or deficient, we can tonify (nourish) its mother and thereby benefit the son. So if there is not enough Fire, corresponding to the Heart, we would strengthen the Wood organ, the Liver, with the proper foods or herbs.

In ancient times these correspondences were made by observing nature and how our bodies worked similarly. In nature the Five Elements can be correlated to the seasons as follows: Wood corresponds to spring, Fire corresponds to summer, Earth corresponds to late summer and the time between seasons, Metal corresponds to autumn, Water corresponds to winter.

There is a useful relationship between food colors and the elements and corresponding body systems. White foods nourish the Lungs; black and dark blue foods nourish the Kidneys; green foods nourish the Liver; yellow and orange foods nourish the Spleen and Stomach; red foods nourish the Heart. Thus, a person with weak digestion (Spleen weakness) should include plenty of the yellow and orange foods, such as sweet potatoes and winter squashes, as these are the color that correspond to the Earth element. Someone with Heart weakness would do well to eat more red foods such as tomatoes and hawthorn berries, as red corresponds to the Fire element.

Another relationship that occurs within the Five Elements is the *control cycle*. (*Refer to Chart 3*.) It goes like this: we take wood, a tree, for example, whose roots invade into the earth; we take earth and build a dam to control water; water puts out the fire; fire melts down the metal; metal makes the ax that cuts the wood. If Wood (Liver) becomes excessive, manifesting as hypertension, red eyes, and headache, we may want to strengthen or tonify the Metal element (Lungs) to control the Wood.

The *creative* and *control cycles* occur as natural phenomena, keeping life in balance. However, when any one of the elements is either too strong or too weak, disharmony results. Keep in mind as you use the Five Elements Theory that there are always exceptions to the rule.

The Five Tastes

The physical sensation of taste has its significance in Chinese Medicine. In Chinese Medicine, it is classified into five flavors, although in the text you will actually find seven. These five tastes are sour, sweet, bitter, pungent and salty. The other two are bland, which falls under the sweet category, and astringent, which goes under the sour category.

When a substance such as a food or an herb goes into the gastrointestinal tract to be digested, the sour taste is said to be absorbed by the Liver and Gall Bladder, the bitter taste by the Heart and Small Intestines, the sweet taste by the Spleen and Stomach, the pungent taste by the Lungs and Large Intestines, and the salty taste by the Kidney and

Bladder. Therefore, foods and herbs with different energies and tastes are assimilated into the body to nourish different organs.

Take the example of someone with digestive difficulties as in a weakness of Spleen and Stomach; he or she often likes to eat sweets. Contrary to Western medicine, in that those with digestive weakness are advised against sweets intake, Chinese Medicine utilizes foods that are actually slightly sweet to strengthen the weakness of Spleen and Stomach, such as yam or winter squash. Thus, consumption of foods with various tastes will benefit those organs that correspond to these tastes.

Pungent is a taste that has functions of dispersing, invigorating, and promoting circulation. Its function of dispersing is mainly used to disperse pathogens from the exterior of the body, such as we see in common colds and flu. Its function of invigorating is to promote circulation of Chi, blood and body fluid. In Chinese Medicine, disease is the result of stagnation, therefore, foods that have this pungent taste will promote and invigorate circulation of the Chi, blood and body fluids. Pathological condition of stagnation can be seen as local pain, irregular menstruation, painful menstruation, edema, tumors, and so on. The pungent taste, because of its dispersing quality also acts to open the pores and promote sweating. This is a way to expel the pathogen from the body. Examples of pungent tasting foods are ginger, garlic and mint.

Sour taste has absorbing, consolidating, and astringent functions. It functions in stopping abnormal discharge of body fluids and substances as in condition of excessive perspiration, diarrhea, seminal emission, spermatorrhea, enuresis and so on. Examples of a sour foods are Chinese sour plum, lemon and vinegar.

Astringent taste falls under the sour taste category and its actions are very similar to that of the sour taste.

Bitter tasting substances have the action of drying dampness and dispersing. Often bitter also clears heat. So bitter aids conditions like dampness and edema. Its function of dispersing obstruction can be utilized in cough due to Chi stagnation and so forth. Examples of bitter tasting food are rhubarb, apricot kernels, and kale.

Salty taste has the function of softening and dissolving hardenings. It also moistens and lubricates the intestines. Body symptoms such as lumps, nodes, masses, cysts and so on can be softened and dissolved by salty substances. Example can be seen in goiter which is treated by seaweed, a representative of salty food. Also, in cases of constipation, one can drink salt water to lubricate the intestines and promote evacuation.

Sweet taste has the action of tonifying, harmonizing and decelerating. In cases of fatigue or deficiency, sweet substances have a reinforcing and strengthening action. Deficiencies may occur in different aspects of the body, such as insufficiency of Chi, blood, Yin or Yang. Specific organs may suffer from weakness also. This is why one is drawn to sweet when he or she is experiencing low energy. Sweet taste is also used to decelerate, which means to relax. It is used in conditions of acute pain to help relax and hence, ease the pain. Sweet foods and herbs can harmonize as an antidote or counter balance undesirable effects from some herbs. Example of sweet tasting foods are yams, corn and rice.

Bland taste falls in under the sweet taste category. It tends to be diuretic, promotes urination and relieves edema. An example of a bland tasting food is pearl barley.

The Eight Differentiations

In order to more clearly understand the energy of the patient and the nature and location of the disease, the Chinese have developed this system of diagnosis. *Internal* and *External* serves to locate the area of disease. *Deficient* and *Excess* determine the relative strength of the patient or the disease. *Cold* and *Hot* give indications of the nature of the individual and/or the pathogens. *Yin* and *Yang* give the overall picture of the condition. Together these eight differentiations can provide an accurate picture of both the individual being treated and the disease at hand. Often there is a mixture of symptoms that can be confusing. These principles provide a basis to better understand seemingly contradictive symptoms. A practitioner of Traditional Chinese Medicine would evaluate these continuum based on the tongue and pulse readings, and the presenting signs and symptoms.

Causes of Disease

In Traditional Chinese Medicine, the cause of disease is said to be of an *external* or *internal* source. Just below the surface of the skin lies a layer of energy that acts as a protective shield. In a healthy person this shield is strong and without gaps, as a barrier of protection should be: impervious to external factors. If, however, there are weak spots in this shield and external factors can penetrate into the body, we have disease. This is part of the immune system. If one's immune system is strong, one does not catch the pathogen. For example, some people have the A.I.D.S. virus and show no symptoms of it; others catch it and die shortly. That is the difference between strong Chi and weak Chi.

In the Chinese perception of disease, external causes of diseases include the following environmental conditions:

cold, heat, summer heat, dryness, dampness, and wind. In Western thinking, we would put viruses and bacteria in this category.

Diseases can also arise as a result of internal factors. These include the emotions: joy (mania), grief, anger, depression, worry, melancholy, and fear. These reflect the mental state induced by one's environment. That in itself does not cause disease. However, when emotions are very intense or long lasting, disharmony or disease can result. Mental attitude is very important for good health. By calming one's mind many physical problems disappear.

An interesting survey done in China on a group of cancer patients showed that 95% had been physically or mentally tortured during the Cultural Revolution (1965-1975). During that harsh period intellectuals were tortured and even husbands and wives betrayed each other for the sake of the Party. You could not trust anyone with your inner most feelings and thoughts. These people built up frustration, depression, and anger; these destructive emotions in turn became cancers. Isolation and inability to express emotions is very destructive to one's health.

So remember the importance of emotional balance in maintaining good health. We must have a channel to release any excessive emotion, be it exercises such a T'ai Chi Ch'uan or Chi Gong, breathing techniques, acupuncture, meditation, or walking. These activities can help to regulate emotions and promote more inner peace.

Other miscellaneous causes of disease would include traumatic injury, stagnant blood or mucus, improper exercise, improper activities, and improper diet. Traumatic injuries would include accidents, incisions, sprains, burns, and animal or insect bites. Stagnancy of the blood and mucus cause blocks in the energy pathways; a good example is tumors.

Either too much or too little exercise can cause disease. Improper activities would include excessive sex, overworking, and overexertion. Excessive sex is particularly injurious to the Kidneys, the storehouse of our Jing. Improper diet could be eating too little for proper nourishment of the body, overeating, or eating too much of the wrong foods, such as too much raw, cold, greasy, or spicy foods.

Overeating is a very common imbalance in this country that causes many diseases. Americans constantly overeat because they do not know how to eat and tend to eat very fast. By slowly chewing one's food properly, the body will tell you when to stop. Also, people reach out to food and use it as an escape. Eating in a relaxed frame of mind is essential to good digestion and assimilation of nutrients.

It has been found in animal experiments that if one group is allowed to eat as much as desired and another group is fasted every second day, the first group has five times more tendency toward spontaneous cancer. An interesting statistic: U.S. leads the world in both protein consumption per person and the incidence of cancer. Protein is needed, but an excessive amount causes problems. An over consumption of meat protein will also result in a high percentage of fat in the diet, another big contributor to disease. Meat companies have led us to believe that we need far more protein than is really healthy. Moderation is essential to good health.

A significant study, conducted from 1983 - 1988, of 6,500 people from 65 counties across China, showed the great impact that regular exercise and a low fat, high fiber diet have on maintaining good health. This was the largest study of its kind done to date. The findings of the China Project on Nutrition, Health and the Environment were published in 1990 as *Diet, Lifestyle and Mortality in China*. This project was under the direction of T. Colin Campbell of Cornell

University, in collaboration with researchers from Oxford University, Chinese Academy of Preventive Medicine, and Chinese Academy of Medical Sciences, both in Beijing. The results suggested that the healthiest diet would contain a minimum of 80 - 90% plant foods. Those in the Chinese countryside who get only about 10 - 15 % of their calories and 7% of their total protein from animal products, had low incidence of heart disease, colon cancer, and osteoporosis. The study showed that when the rural dweller moved to the city and adopted the city lifestyle and higher fat diet (30%), diseases increased.

The Western approach to diseases is to kill the bacteria and suppress the symptoms, thus driving the disease deeper into the body. The Chinese way supports the body and lets it do the killing of the pathogen. Supporting the body with tonification reinforces the body's healing energy. Remember that the body can heal itself if given the proper chance. We may need to give it a little help through nutritional measures or herbal medicines.

Fasting or light eating is sometimes recommended during an illness, such as a cold, so as not to detract from the body's healing by having to digest heavy foods. In many traditions throughout the world, a thin, soupy grain porridge is given during illness. This is very easily digested, thus, the body can draw on its resources to heal. The antibiotic route, on the other hand, weakens the immune system, makes one more prone to illness, causes the immune system to become lazy, and generally interferes with the natural healing process.

There are many possible supportive measures through food and herbs that can be taken. In many instances, along with supporting the body we also need to concurrently detoxify or sedate it. This is the Chinese approach to disease. For cancer patients in some hospitals in China, doctors combine the killing aspects of chemotherapy and radiation with the supportive measures of Traditional Chinese Medicine, including proper diet, herbs, Chi Gong exercises and acupuncture. This has produced a longer life expectancy than the conventional killing approach alone. Then some hospitals treat cancer patients solely with Chinese medicine; this group shows the longest life expectancy with many total remissions

Prevention of Disease

As we increase our awareness of health, we can hopefully maintain a state of balance within the body, and become more responsible for our health. Too often we suffer from our inappropriate actions and thoughts. Chinese Nutrition stresses the prevention of disease. In *The Yellow Emperor's Classic of Internal Medicine*, written 2000-3000 years ago, it was said, *A doctor who treats a disease after it has happened is a mediocre doctor, but a doctor who treats a disease before it happens is a superior doctor.* Doctors were considered to be teachers who taught their patients how to be healthy and spiritually upright. Success was measured by vibrant health. We as individuals can choose to be one kind of doctor or the other.

Traditionally, herbs have been used to preserve good health, and prevent disease. Many of the tonifying herbs are used for this purpose over a long period of time. The tonic herbs are further categorized into Yin, Yang, Blood and Chi tonics, and lend themselves well to preparations with foods, such as soups, stews and porridges. Incorporating the appropriate herbs into the diet on a regular basis can provide great benefit to health.

The use of herbs as food has a long history in China. The first Chinese Materia Medica, *Shen-Nong Herbal Classic*, categorizes herbs into three groups. The First group was called *food herbs*, which were eaten as a part of the diet for general nourishment, for maintenance of health, and prevention of disease. The Taoist hermits called these herbs *immortal foods* and described them as producing effects that *rejuvenate health, prolong life, restore youth, and increase clarity.* They often used them as the main part of their diet, along with some fruits, nuts and seeds. Later sections of this book describe some of these *food herbs*. For extensive details on *food herbs* and recipes, we refer you to the Bibliography, and in particular, *101 Vegetarian Delights* by Lily Chuang and Cathy McNease and *Chinese Vegetarian Delights* by Lily Chuang.

The other two groups of herbs were called *medicinal herbs,* which are dispensed to each patient in an individual formula based on ones constitution, environment and medical condition, by an Oriental Medical professional.

Prevention of disease includes proper nutrition, emotional balance, proper exercise, as well as nourishing our spirit. As we nourish body, mind, and spirit we maintain a state of balance. Preventative maintenance is the most sensible route to take. As The Yellow Emperor states: *The sages of ancient times emphasized not the treatment of disease, but rather the prevention of its occurrence. To administer medicine to disease which has already developed and to suppress revolts which have already begun is comparable to the behavior of one who begins to dig a well after he has become thirsty or one who begins to forge weapons after he has engaged in battle. Would these actions not be too late?*

Guidelines for a Balanced Diet

As every body is unique, there will always be variations according to individual needs. A few basic guidelines, however, are appropriate as we seek a way of eating that creates balance and harmony. Frame of mind is of utmost importance at mealtime; relax and slowly chew your food for optimal digestion and assimilation. The dinner table is not the place to discuss the day's problems. Chewing is a major part of digestion. Remember, your stomach does not have teeth. Digestion, particularly of the starches, begins in the mouth. Foods that are difficult to thoroughly masticate, such as sesame seeds, should be ground before eating. Fruits digest quickly, while meats and proteins will take more time to digest.

The best ways of preparing foods are steaming, stir frying in water, stewing (boiling, as in soups), or baking. Steaming leaves the food in its most natural state, while baking creates more heat and would be the best method for cold conditions. Even the best quality oils become hard to digest when heated. So, if oil is desired, put it on after the food is cooked.

Foods should be eaten in their wholeness, when possible. Only peel fruits or vegetables if the peel is hard to digest or contaminated with chemical sprays. Search out organically grown foods to avoid the toxic chemical residues of commercial growing processes. To clean foods thoroughly one may wash them in salt water. Also avoid irradiated foods and microwave ovens, if possible. The best utensils for cooking in are glass, earthenware, or stainless steel. One should avoid cooking in aluminum or copper; these metals can easily leach into the food.

One's diet should follow the seasons, eating what grows locally. Nature has the perfect plan in providing the appropriate foods for the given season. The fruits and vegetables that ripen in the summertime tend to be on the cooling side. In wintertime we will tend toward a more warming diet. Also, one should eat a wide variety of foods for good balance.

Most vegetables should be at least lightly cooked as raw vegetables tend to be difficult to digest. Foods should never be eaten cold because cold foods *put out the dige*stive *fire*, so to say. This is particularly upsetting to the female menstrual cycle as the stomach sits right beside the liver which is responsible for storing blood. Cooling off the stomach can lead to a stagnant blood condition and a difficult menstrual period. Frozen foods, such as ice cream, are a very unhealthy item, as well as iced drinks. Neither should we consume foods that are so hot that they burn the mouth or stomach.

It is best to stop eating before the *full* point. Also, eating just before retiring is not a good idea. One should take the last meal at least 3 hours before going to bed. This will not only result in better digestion, but also a more restful sleep. Late eating also tends to easily be stored as unwanted pounds. One should wake up with a good appetite for breakfast. This is the meal that provides us with the fuel or energy for much of the day, so make this a very nutritious meal.

Nuts and seeds contain a large proportion of oil and should be eaten as fresh as possible and kept refrigerated. Because most people do not chew nuts well, grinding them into powder makes them easier to digest.

Beans should be soaked prior to cooking for at least a few hours; always discard the soak water and cook them in fresh water. The small beans like lentils and peas tend to be easier to digest than the large beans like limas or kidney beans. For a person with particularly weak digestion it is best to cook grains *soupy*, with additional water and cooking time. You may use up to 10 parts water per 1 part of grain.

Always avoid highly processed foods and keep meals as simple as possible. A balanced diet would consist of the following on a regular basis:
WHOLE GRAINS including rice, millet, barley, wheat, oats, corn, rye, quinoa, amaranth, etc. This group of foods will account for about **40% of the diet.**
FRESHLY PREPARED VEGETABLES including dark

leafy greens, cabbage, broccoli, celery, root vegetables, etc. This group of foods will account for about **40% of the diet.**
FRESH FRUITS will be consumed when in season, and generally **no more than 10% of the diet.** Fruits can be a great snack or sweet treat.
LEGUMES / SEEDS / NUTS including peas, beans, tofu, peanuts, lentils, sunflower seeds, almonds, walnuts, etc. This will account for about **10 - 20% of the vegetarian diet and a lesser portion of the meat inclusive diet**
ANIMAL PRODUCTS including dairy foods, meat, fish, poultry, and eggs. If one chooses to include these foods in the diet, they should occupy **no more than 10% of the diet.** Attempt to locate growers that do not use drugs or inhumane practices on the animals.
SEAWEEDS including *nori, wakame, dulse, kombu, hiziki,* and *arame.* This is a valuable mineral source, consumed in **small amounts** (a small handful dry), and of particular value to those vegetarians who refrain from eating dairy foods.

Avoid as strictly as possible the following: chemical preservatives, additives, colorings and flavorings, M.S.G., fried or greasy foods, coffee, ice cream and excessive sugar consumption.

The USDA recently adopted *a Food Pyramid* as an alternative to the out-dated *Basic Four Food Groups.* It is very similar to the food group proportions used in Chinese Nutrition. Grains, beans, vegetables and fruits constitute the base of the pyramid and majority of the diet, while meat and dairy foods, eaten in small proportions, are at the top. Perhaps this change shows the realization of more Americans that we need to make changes in our dietary habits and ways of looking at food.

SECTION

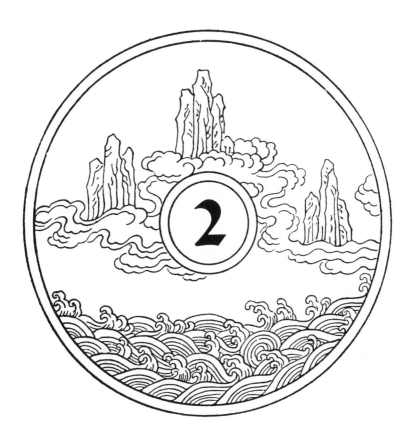

Foods

VEGETABLES

ALFALFA SPROUT

Nature / Taste: cool and slightly bitter

Actions: benefits spleen and stomach, dispels dampness, lubricates intestines

Conditions: swelling, constipation, skin lesions

Folk Remedies:

1. SWELLING - boil tea and drink 3 times daily.

2. CONSTIPATION - eat raw alfalfa sprouts.

3. SKIN LESIONS - apply mashed alfalfa sprouts; change poultice 3-4 times daily.

ASPARAGUS

Nature / Taste: cool, sweet and bitter

Actions: clears heat, detoxifies, promotes blood circulation, clears lungs

Conditions: constipation, cancer, hypertension, high blood cholesterol, arteriosclerosis, bronchitis

Folk Remedies:

1. HIGH CHOLESTEROL, HYPERTENSION, AND ARTERIOSCLEROSIS - drink 1 glass daily of blender-made asparagus juice, including the pulp; add 1 teaspoon of honey.

2. BREAST CANCER - boil asparagus with dandelions; drink the liquid and apply the solids to the area.

3. CONSTIPATION - eat asparagus with cabbage, lightly steamed.

BAMBOO SHOOT

Nature / Taste: cool and sweet

Actions: strengthens the stomach, relieves food retention, resolves mucus, promotes diuresis, cuts or emulsifies fats, relieves alcohol intoxication, promotes measles

Conditions: diabetes, indigestion, stomach distention and fullness due to greasy food, diarrhea, dysentery, rectal prolapse, edema

Contraindications: Not to be used after giving birth as they may trigger the cleansing of an old illness, manifesting in skin lesions.

Folk Remedies:
1. DIARRHEA, DYSENTERY, AND RECTAL PROLAPSE - cook bamboo shoots with rice.

2. SWELLING DUE TO KIDNEY, HEART, OR LIVER DISEASE - drink tea of bamboo shoots and winter melon rind.

3. DIABETES - blend bamboo shoots and celery juice, warm up and drink 1 cup twice daily. Eat plenty of bamboo shoots.

4. STOMACH DISTENTION AND FULLNESS - make tea from bamboo shoots, ginger, and orange peel, and drink.

BEET

Nature / Taste: cool and sweet

Actions: nourishes blood, tonifies the heart, calms the spirit, lubricates the intestines, cleanses the liver

Conditions: anemia, heart weakness, irritability, restlessness, habitual constipation, herpes, constipation, liver intoxication from drugs or alcohol

Contraindications: Not for someone with a history of kidney stones because of the oxalic acid content.

Folk Remedies:

1. CONSTIPATION - make beet soup, or combine beets with cabbage.

2. BLOOD DEFICIENCY - cook beets with black beans and peanuts.

3. LIVER CLEANSING - drink beet top tea, or combine with dandelions and make tea.

4. HERPES - do a 3 day fast with vegetable broth* and beet top tea.

Basic vegetable broth for detoxification can be made by simmering carrots and carrot tops, celery, dandelions, asparagus, and squash.

BELL PEPPER

Nature / Taste: slightly warm, pungent and sweet

Actions: strengthens stomach, improves appetite, promotes blood circulation, removes stagnant food, reduces swelling

Conditions: indigestion, decreased appetite, swelling, frostbite, food retention

Folk Remedies:

1. INDIGESTION AND FOOD RETENTION - make green pepper tea.

2. FROSTBITE - wash affected area in bell pepper and cinnamon tea, and drink the tea.

3. DECREASED APPETITE AND ANOREXIA - mix bell pepper with black pepper and dry fry (no oil).Or lightly fry chunks of bell pepper with oil.

BOK CHOY

Nature / Taste: cool, pungent and sweet

Actions: clears heat, lubricates the intestines, removes stagnant food, quenches thirst, promotes digestion

Conditions: food retention, constipation, indigestion, diabetes

Folk Remedies:

1. FOOD RETENTION - boil tea or soup from bok choy and orange peel.

2. INDIGESTION - eat pickled bok choy.

3. CONSTIPATION - cook bok choy with beets.

4. THIRST - drink bok choy and cucumber juice.

BROCCOLI

Nature / Taste: cool and sweet

Actions: clears heat, promotes diuresis, brightens eyes, clears summer heat problems. This vegetable is weak in action.

Conditions: conjunctivitis, nearsightedness, difficult urination, irritability

Folk Remedies:

1. CLEAR HEAT - eat lightly steamed broccoli.

2. CONJUNCTIVITIS - drink carrot and broccoli tea.

3. URINARY DIFFICULTY - combine broccoli with Chinese cabbage and make soup.

BURDOCK ROOT (GOBO)

Nature / Taste: cool, pungent and bitter

Actions: clears heat, dispels wind, brightens vision

Conditions: common cold of the wind-heat type, sore throat, measles, conjunctivitis, mumps

Contraindications: Not to be used in cases of diarrhea.

Folk Remedies:
1. CONJUNCTIVITIS - boil tea and expose eyes to the steam then drink the tea.

2. COMMON COLD AND MEASLES - drink burdock tea and sweat.

3. MUMPS - make burdock and dandelion tea, apply locally and drink the tea.

CABBAGE (RED OR GREEN)

Nature / Taste: cool and sweet

Actions: clears heat, lubricates intestines, stops cough

Conditions: constipation, whooping cough, hot flashes, common colds, frostbite

Folk Remedies:
1. COMMON COLD - take 1/4 head cabbage and 3 green onions, boil 10 minutes and drink the liquid, and sweat.

2. WHOOPING COUGH - make cabbage tea and add 2 teaspoons honey to lubricate the lungs (or add apricot kernel).

3. FROSTBITE - wash the area in warm cabbage and green onion tea.

CARROT

Nature / Taste: cool, sweet and pungent

Actions: clears heat, detoxifies, strengthens all internal organs, benefits the eyes, relieves measles, lubricates the intestines, promotes digestion

Folk Remedies:

1. NIGHT BLINDNESS - drink lukewarm carrot juice.

2. DIPHTHERIA WITH SORE THROAT - drink carrot top tea.

3. INDIGESTION - make carrot tea and add a teaspoon of brown sugar or maltose.

4. MEASLES - make tea from carrots, water chestnut, and cilantro to induce eruption. It goes away after completely erupting.

5. SKIN LESIONS OR EYE WEAKNESS - make tea or juice from carrots and carrot tops.

6. CANCER - to prevent, cook 1/2 stick carrot with Chinese black mushrooms and consume daily. Also drink carrot top tea.

CAULIFLOWER

Nature / Taste: cool and sweet

Actions: lubricates the intestines, strengthens spleen. This vegetable is weak in action.

Conditions: constipation, weak digestion

Folk Remedies:

1. WEAK DIGESTION - eat lightly steamed cauliflower with bell pepper and celery.

2. CONSTIPATION - eat raw cauliflower in salad.

CELERY

Nature / Taste: cool , sweet and slightly bitter

Actions: tonifies kidney, stops bleeding, strengthens spleen and stomach, clears heat, lowers blood pressure, promotes diuresis, benefits blood

Folk Remedies:

1. HIGH BLOOD PRESSURE (HYPERTENSION) - eat celery regularly; drink 3 cups lightly boiled celery juice daily. Or drink lukewarm celery juice on an empty stomach daily.

2. DIABETES - drink 3 cups lightly boiled celery juice daily. Or combine celery, yam and pumpkin to make vegetable pie.

3. WHOOPING COUGH - lightly steam celery juice, add a pinch of salt, take a warm glassful at 5 A.M. and at 7 P.M., three days in a row.

4. INSOMNIA - take celery and beet tops tea in the evening, 2 hours prior to bed time.

CHARD

Nature / Taste: neutral and sweet

Actions: clears heat, detoxifies, benefits blood

Conditions: dysentery, boils, skin lesions

Folk Remedies

1. DYSENTERY - make a tea from chard and dandelion greens.

2. BOILS - apply external mixed with aloe vera juice.

CHINESE CABBAGE (NAPA CABBAGE)

Nature / Taste: cold and sweet

Actions: clears heat, lubricates intestines, promotes urination, diaphoretic

Conditions: irritability, restlessness, constipation, difficulty urinating

Folk Remedies:

1. CONSTIPATION OR DIFFICULTY URINATING - make Chinese cabbage soup.

2. COMMON COLD (WIND-COLD TYPE) - mix Chinese cabbage and ginger, simmer into tea, and sweat.

CHINESE CHIVE

Nature / Taste: warm and pungent

Actions: tonifies kidneys and sexual functions, removes dampness, warms up coldness

Conditions: cold stomachache, leukorrhea, diarrhea, bedwetting, wet dreams, absences of menstrual period

Folk Remedies:

1. For the above conditions, boil Chinese chive tea for 25-30 minutes.

2. WEAK SEXUAL FUNCTIONS - cook Chinese chives with black beans, black sesame seeds, walnuts, sour plums, and 2 tsp. honey. Make into a paste and take 1 Tbsp. 3 times daily.

CILANTRO LEAF (CHINESE PARSLEY)

Nature / Taste : slightly cool* and pungent

Actions: promotes sweating, strengthens digestion, promotes Chi flow

Conditions: measles, common cold, indigestion, lack of appetite, chest and stomach fullness

Folk Remedies:

1. MEASLES - drink cilantro and mint tea to induce eruptions.

2. COMMON COLD OF THE WIND COLD TYPE - drink cilantro and ginger tea.

3. COMMON COLD OF THE WIND HEAT TYPE - drink cilantro and mint tea.

4. CHI STAGNATION - drink cilantro and orange peel tea. *CILANTRO SEEDS (CORIANDER) are slightly warm and beneficial to digestion.*

CORN

Nature / Taste: cool and sweet

Actions: stops bleeding, promotes diuresis, benefits gall bladder, lowers blood pressure, clears heat, detoxifies

Conditions: difficult urination, gallstones, hepatitis, jaundice, hypertension, heart disease

Folk Remedies:

1. HYPERTENSION, JAUNDICE, AND GALLSTONES - eat corn regularly and drink fresh cornsilk tea.

2. DETOXIFY AND CLEAR HEAT - drink cornsilk and dandelion tea.

3. SWELLING OR DIFFICULTY URINATING - drink cornsilk and pearl barley tea.

4. HIGH BLOOD PRESSURE - drink cornsilk and chrysanthemum tea.

5. BLOODY URINE - drink corn and lotus root tea.

CUCUMBER

Nature / Taste: cool, sweet and bland (peels are bitter)

Actions: clears heat, quenches thirst, relieves irritability, promotes diuresis

Conditions: swelling of the extremities, jaundice, diarrhea, epilepsy, sore throat, conjunctivitis

Contraindications: Eating cucumbers to excess will cause dampness. Cucumber seeds are difficult to digest.

Folk Remedies:

1. SWELLING OF THE EXTREMITIES AND JAUN-DICE - boil tea from cucumber skins.

2. DIARRHEA - use 2 teaspoons of dried cucumber meal mixed with rice porridge.

3. EPILEPSY - boil tea from cucumber vines.

4. HOT, SCRATCHY, OR SWOLLEN (PUFFY) EYES - apply grated cucumber packs to closed eyes; leave on 20 minutes.

DAIKON RADISH (WHITE CARROT)

Nature / Taste: cool, pungent and sweet

Actions: removes stagnant food, moistens lungs, resolves mucus, quenches thirst, relieves alcohol intoxication

Conditions: bronchitis, sore throat, dry cough, coughing of blood, painful urination, excess of mucus, alcohol intoxication, food retention

Folk Remedies:

1. BRONCHITIS OR SORE THROAT - make daikon juice and add 2 drops of ginger juice; drink 1 cup lukewarm, 3 times daily.

2. DRY COUGH WITH YELLOW SPUTUM - take warm daikon and water chestnut juice with 1 tsp. honey.

3. BURNS - apply grated daikon alone or mixed with aloe vera gel.

4. ALCOHOL INTOXICATION - drink daikon juice before and after the alcohol.

Contraindication: Not to be consumed with ginseng root because they go opposite directions in the body.

DANDELION GREENS

Nature / Taste: cool, bitter and slightly sweet

Actions: clears heat, detoxifies, anti-tumor, benefits liver function, promotes the flow of bile, diuretic

Conditions: toxic skin lesions, bug bites, poison oak blisters, conjunctivitis, liver heat rising, beginning stages of common cold

Folk Remedies:

1. TOXIC SKIN LESIONS - apply crushed, fresh leaves; change poultice hourly.

2. CONJUNCTIVITIS (LIVER HEAT RISING) - make tea or juice.

3. COMMON COLD - make tea from fresh dandelions (the whole plant), mint, and licorice.

4. BREAST LUMPS AND TUMORS - apply dandelion and ginger poultices.

Dandelion has been found to be extremely effective in inhibiting bacteria, virus, and fungus. It is considered to be a natural anti-biotic similar in action to goldenseal root (Hydrastis canadensis).

EGGPLANT

Nature / Taste: cool and sweet

Actions: relieves pain, promotes diuresis, reduces swelling, removes blood stagnation

Conditions: abdominal pain, dysentery, hot diarrhea, painful urination, frostbite, canker sores, snake and scorpion bites, anal bleeding, hepatitis, jaundice

Contraindications: Not to be used for cold type problems.

Folk Remedies:
1. BITES - apply fresh to absorb toxins.

2. JAUNDICE AND HEPATITIS - eat eggplant and rice 3 times daily for 1 week.

3. SWELLING AND EDEMA - dry the eggplant and grind to a meal; take 1 teaspoon in warm water 3 times daily.

4. FROSTBITE - soak area in eggplant tea.

5. CANKER SORES - charcoal eggplant and apply locally.

GARLIC

Nature / Taste: hot and pungent

Actions: anti-viral, anti-fungal, detoxifies meat and seafood, kills worms, removes stagnant food and stagnant blood, reduces abscess

Conditions: cancer, high blood cholesterol, infections, diarrhea, dysentery, vomiting, and coughing of blood

Contraindications: Not to be used with hot or dry eye disorders, mouth sores or tongue ulcers.

Folk Remedies:

1. VAGINAL INFECTIONS - boil a bulb of garlic, cool to lukewarm, then douche with the liquid.

2. COUGHING OR VOMITING OF BLOOD - apply crushed, peeled, raw garlic to the soles of both feet at the depression behind the ball of the foot, also known as *rushing spring* point (KIDNEY 1); change the poultice every 4 hours.

3. DYSENTERY - mash 3-5 cloves of raw garlic, mix with warm water; drink every 2 hours.

4. VOMITING - cook together a bulb of garlic and 3 slices ginger; mix with a teaspoon of honey and some water.

5. ANTIDOTE FOR CRAB POISONING - cook garlic with crabs or other sea foods.

6. EARACHE OR EAR INFECTION- put a few drops of garlic oil or juice in ear several times daily.

7. INTESTINAL WORMS - eat cooked garlic on an empty stomach; resume eating 3 hours later.

GREEN BEAN

Nature / Taste: warm and sweet

Actions: warms spleen and stomach, descends Chi, tonifies kidneys, benefits Chi

Conditions: burping, chest fullness and discomfort, whooping cough, hernia in children, chronic diarrhea, back pain due to kidney weakness

Folk Remedies:

1. WHOOPING COUGH - boil 1/2 cup green beans and 6 grams licorice in 1 1/2 cups water; boil down to 1 cup and add 2 of teaspoons honey. Drink the liquid.

2. CHRONIC DIARRHEA - steam green beans with rice.

3. HERNIA IN CHILDREN - Dry fry green beans with fennel and then grind into powder. Take 1/2 tsp. each time, 3 times daily with lukewarm water. Also can be applied as a paste (green beans and fennel) to the navel with black pepper.

4. BACK PAIN - make soup with green beans, black beans, and azuki beans and a pinch of cinnamon powder.

KALE

Nature / Taste: warm and slightly bitter

Actions: strengthens stomach, stops pains, promotes regrowth of tissue

Conditions: stomach or duodenal ulcers

Folk Remedies:

1. ULCERS - take 1/2 glass warm kale juice before each meal.

LETTUCE

Nature / Taste: neutral and bland*

Actions: invigorates Chi, removes stagnation, reduces swelling, softens hardening. This vegetable is mild in action.

Conditions: skin lesions, abdominal pain, breast abscess, postpartum abdominal pain due to blood stagnation

Folk Remedies:
1. SKIN LESIONS, INSECT BITES, SORES WITH PUS - apply mashed lettuce, changing poultice 3 times daily; and drink 1 cup of lukewarm lettuce juice, 3 times daily.

2. BREAST ABSCESS - make poultice and juice with dandelions. Drink the juice and apply with gauze pad externally.

The more bitter varieties of lettuce like ROMAINE or ENDIVE are cool and drying.

LOTUS ROOT

Nature / Taste: cool and sweet

Actions: very healing, clears heat, quenches thirst, relieves irritability, stops bleeding, strengthens the stomach, promotes diuresis, cools the blood

Conditions: difficult urination, vomiting blood, nosebleed, blood in stool or urine, hypertension, gastritis, colitis

Folk Remedies:
1. NOSEBLEED AND HYPERTENSION - drink lotus root juice daily.

2. GASTRITIS AND COLITIS - drink diluted lotus root juice.

3. VOMITING OR DEFECATING BLOOD - cook 1/2 c. of lotus root starch with 1/2 c. of rice porridge until jelly like consistency; consume while lukewarm.

4. BLOOD IN THE URINE - make tea of lotus root and bamboo leaves.

MUSHROOM (BUTTON)

Nature / Taste: slightly cool and sweet

Actions: induces measle eruptions, detoxifies, improves appetite, stops diarrhea, resolves phlegm, anti-tumor

Conditions: infectious hepatitis, measles, diarrhea, cough with copious mucus, low appetite

Folk Remedies:
1. INFECTIOUS HEPATITIS, LEUKOCYTOPENIA - take button mushrooms in the diet or in tea.

2. MEASLES - boil tea from button mushrooms and drink one cup 3 times daily. Or, cook with poi and drink the broth.

MUSHROOM (GANODERMA, LING ZHI)

Nature / Taste: warm and bland

Actions: nourish the heart, calm the spirit, fortify the Chi and blood

Conditions: heart Chi deficiency, blood deficiency leading to insomnia, excessive dreaming, anxiety, restlessness, fatigue; coughs, asthma, high cholesterol, high blood pressure, coronary heart disease, chronic hepatitis, low white blood cell production.

Folk Remedies
1. HIGH BLOOD PRESSURE, HIGH CHOLESTEROL - Ling Zhi mushroom is usually consumed in powder or tea form on a daily routine.

2. CHRONIC HEPATITIS - make tea from Ling Zhi and licorice root.

3. CHRONIC BRONCHITIS - make a tea of Ling Zhi and lily bulbs.

4. ALLERGIC ASTHMA - make tea of Ling Zhi, basil, and peppermint.

5. ALLERGIC RHINITIS - concentrate the Ling Zhi tea, strain through filter paper, then wash nose with the tea.

These are also known as REISHI MUSHROOMS.

MUSHROOM (SHITAKE , BLACK)

Nature / Taste: neutral and sweet

Actions: strengthens stomach, promotes healing, lowers blood pressure, detoxifies, anti-tumor, lowers cholesterol

Conditions: tumor, diabetes, hypertension, slow healing, high blood pressure, high cholesterol

Folk Remedies:
1. TUMORS - boil tea from black mushrooms and drink 3 times daily, continuously. This can also be used as a preventative to stomach and cervical cancer. Used post surgery, this remedy can prevent metastasis (spreading) of the tumor cells.

2. TO CLEAN TOXINS IN THE INTESTINES - soak some Chinese black mushrooms, blend with the soak water; heat like soup and take on an empty stomach. One can also add a little ginger.

These are also referred to as CHINESE MUSHROOMS.

MUSHROOM (WHITE)

Nature / Taste: cold and sweet

Actions: clears summer heat, lowers blood pressure, anti-tumor, detoxifies

Conditions: hypertension, summer irritability and other summer heat problems, tumors

Contraindications: White mushrooms should not be used by those with skin problems, allergies or cold stomach.

Folk Remedies:

1. HIGH BLOOD CHOLESTEROL OR HYPERTENSION - use white mushrooms and cornsilk, and make soup or tea regularly.

2. TUMORS - make mushroom soup or tea daily and drink 3 cups daily.

3. SUMMER HEAT PROBLEMS - eat raw mushrooms in salad.

This is the common supermarket variety of mushroom. Seek out ones that are grown without chemicals.

MUSTARD GREEN

Nature / Taste: warm and pungent

Actions: relieves common colds, promotes diuresis, dissolves mucus, strengthens and lubricates intestines, ventilates lungs, increases appetite

Conditions: difficulty urinating, coughing of blood, dysentery, sore throat, loss of voice, copious white sputum

Folk Remedies:

1. DIFFICULTY URINATING - make tea from fresh mustard greens and drink frequently.

2. COUGHING OF BLOOD - make raw mustard greens juice, mix with some lukewarm water and gradually drink.

3. DYSENTERY - charcoal mustard plant roots and grind into meal. Mix 6 ounces of meal with water and add 1 teaspoon of honey; drink 2 times daily.

4. COMMON COLD (WIND COLD TYPE) - drink tea of mustard greens, cilantro and green onions and try to sweat.

5. COPIOUS WHITE SPUTUM - drink mustard seed tea.

ONION (OR LEEK)

Nature / Taste: warm and pungent

Actions: promotes sweating, resolves phlegm, diuretic

Conditions: common cold, acute or chronic sinus infection, upper respiratory infection, allergies, difficulty urinating, intestinal worms, certain types of boils and lesions

Folk Remedies:
1. COMMON COLD - make tea from chopped onion and a couple slices of fresh ginger root. Or just eat the onion.

2. COMMON COLD AND SINUS CONGESTION IN INFANTS - rub onion juice on baby's upper lip, under the nose, or vaporize the room with steam from onion tea.

3. CHRONIC OR ACUTE SINUS INFECTION - before bedtime rinse nasal passages with saline solution. Then extract onion juice and soak 2 cotton balls in it. Then insert into nostril, one at a time and leave there for 5 minutes each.

4. COUGH, MUCUS, AND UPPER RESPIRATORY INFECTION - put slices of onion over the nose like a mask and inhale the aroma for 30 minutes. Or steam the sliced onion and apply warm as a poultice to the chest area; cover to keep warm and leave on for 20 - 30 minutes.

5. DIFFICULTY URINATING - mash onion and steam it; then apply poultice to the abdomen below the navel (CV4) as a hot compress.

6. INTESTINAL WORMS IN CHILDREN - mash onion and mix with 1-2 T. Sesame oil and eat on an empty stomach twice a day for 3 consecutive days.

7. BOILS - mash and mix with vinegar and apply to lesions

The properties of ONION would also apply to LEEK.

PARSLEY

Nature / Taste: slightly warm and pungent

Actions: promotes digestion, removes stagnant food, regulates flow of Chi, induces measle eruption, diuretic

Conditions: food retention, indigestion, stomach and abdominal fullness, measles, seafood or meat poisoning

Contraindications: Over consumption of parsley is not beneficial for the eyes.

Folk Remedies:

1. BREAST ABSCESS - make juice from 1/2 pound parsley; divide into 3 portions to be taken with warm wine.

2. MEASLES - make parsley tea; drink and mix the tea with wine to be used as a wash, externally to induce eruption.

3. FOOD RETENTION, INDIGESTION, AND FULLNESS - make tea of parsley, hawthorn berries, daikon radish, and unsprayed, dried orange peels.

PARSLEY is a strong food that is eaten in small amounts. Seek naturally grown parsley, if possible.

PARSNIP

Nature / Taste: warm and pungent

Actions: promotes sweating, dispels wind and dampness, relieves pain, stops bleeding (when charred)*

Conditions: common cold of the wind cold type, headache, muscle ache, dizziness, arthritis, tetanus

Folk Remedies:
1. COMMON COLD (WIND-DAMP-COLD TYPE) - make parsnip and ginger tea.

2. ARTHRITIS OF THE WIND- COLD TYPE - combine parsnip, cinnamon, black pepper, and dry ginger to make tea, and drink. Externally apply either mashed, fresh jalepeno pepper or dry jalepeno mixed with some ginger tea.
Charred parsnips used as tea are used to stop bleeding such as coughing blood or nosebleeds.

POTATO

Nature / Taste: cool and sweet

Actions: relieves ulcer pain, strengthens spleen, harmonizes stomach, tonifies Chi, lubricates intestines, promotes diuresis, heals inflammations

Conditions: stomach and duodenal ulcers, constipation, eczema, skin lesions, swelling, small physical stature.

Contraindications: Do not eat sprouted or green potatoes because they are poisonous.

Folk Remedies:
1. ULCER PAIN OR CONSTIPATION - make raw potato juice in the blender, mix with a small amount of honey; take 2 tablespoons every morning on an empty stomach. Make fresh daily.

2. ECZEMA OR OTHER DAMP, EXUDING SORES - apply raw grated potato locally with gauze, change every 3 hours.

3. GENITAL ECZEMA - apply raw grated potato at night; change 6 times; repeat for 3 days.

4. SWELLING - make tea of grated potato and cucumber.

PUMPKIN (AND WINTER SQUASH)

WINTER SQUASHES are the hard skin varieties like acorn, butternut, buttercup, spaghetti, and kobocha.

Nature / Taste: cool and sweet

Actions: dispels dampness, reduces fever, relieves pain, stabilizes hyperactive fetus, stops dysentery, benefits diabetes; the seeds kill worms and parasites

Conditions: dysentery, diabetes, ulcerations of the lower extremities, eczema, stomachache, the feeling of *steaming bones**, antidote for opium

Folk Remedies:

1. BURNS - apply fresh pumpkin alone or mixed with aloe vera gel.

2. LOWER LIMB ULCERATIONS - apply dried pumpkin meal.

3. INTESTINAL WORMS - take 1 teaspoon pumpkin seed meal 3 times daily on an empty stomach.

4. CHILDHOOD VOMITING - make tea from the pumpkin stem and top *cap*.

5. BREAST CANCER - charcoal the *cap* and grind to powder. Take 1 teaspoon of the powder in 1 shot of rice wine 2 times daily. The alcohol is a useful agent for increasing

circulation and removing stagnancy. The tumor is considered to be some type of stagnant blood, Chi, or mucus.

6. HYPERACTIVE FETUS - take 1 teaspoon pumpkin ash in sweet rice porridge.

7. DIABETES - eat a slice of pumpkin with every meal or bake pie with pumpkin, yam, and potato.

The sensation of heat deep in the body as if steam in the bones is part of a condition of Yin exhaustion in the body, along with insomnia, irritability, flushed cheeks, heat, especially severe in late afternoon or evenings, night sweats, thirst, feverish sensation in palms and soles.

SCALLION (GREEN ONION)

Nature / Taste: hot*and pungent

Actions: expels external pathogens, dispels wind and cold, induces sweating, anti-viral, and anti-bacterial

Conditions: common cold, nasal congestion, measles, abscesses, arthritis of the *cold type*

Contraindication: Not to be used for the *heat type* arthritis. Not to be used for heat stages of common cold, characterized by fever, extreme thirst, and yellow sputum.

Folk Remedies:
1. COMMON COLD - make tea by lightly boiling scallions for 5 minutes. Basil and scallion tea is also good.

2. MEASLES - drink scallion tea and apply raw, mashed scallions to the navel to draw out the measles.

3. ABSCESSES - mix raw scallions with egg white and apply; change poultice every 4 hours.

4. ARTHRITIS PAIN - make scallion tea and soak painful
area; apply mashed, cooked scallions to painful area. Scallion and clove tea is also good to drink.

The white part is hot, the green part is warm.

SEAWEED

Nature / Taste: cold and salty

Actions: softens hardenings, clears heat, detoxifies, benefits
the thyroid gland, neutralizes radioactive material, benefits
the lymphatic system, promotes diuresis, provides many
minerals

Conditions: swollen lymph glands, goiters, cough, lung
abscess with thick, yellow, odoriferous mucus, edema,
beriberi, fibroid tumors, cystic breasts, nodules, lumps, cancer, low thyroid

Folk Remedies:

1. GOITER - make soup from dried (preferably green)
orange peel, carrots, and seaweed.

2. LYMPH TUBERCULOSIS - incorporate seaweeds into
the diet for at least 2 months.

3. COUGH AND LUNG ABSCESS - powder seaweed and
mix with honey; these can be rolled into pills.

4. LUMPS, NODULES, AND TUMORS - make tea from
seaweed, peach kernel and green orange peels to take internally. Externally, make poultice of seaweed, ginger, and
dandelion and apply locally.

*There are many varieties of seaweed that can be easily incor-
porated into soups, stir fry dishes, etc. A delicious and healthful
appetizer can be made with soaked hiziki or arame (looks like
thin black noodles), a little soy sauce, honey, and rice vinegar.
The variety of seaweed that would be the least cold is nori.*

SNOW PEA

Nature / Taste: cold and sweet

Actions: strengthens middle warmer, detoxifies, relieves vomiting, promotes diuresis, relieves belching, stops dysentery, aids lactation, quenches thirst

Conditions: chronic diarrhea, dysentery, difficulty urinating, lower abdominal distention and fullness, diabetes, lactostasis, vomiting

Folk Remedies:
1. DIABETES - cook snow peas, then blend juice; take 1/2 cup 2 times daily.

2. HYPERTENSION - make juice from fresh snow peas; take 1/2 cup 2 times daily.

3. DIARRHEA - cook snow peas in sweet rice and take it every meal until relieved.

4. LACTOSTASIS - consume steamed snow peas frequently.

SOYBEAN SPROUT

Nature / Taste: cool and sweet

Actions: promotes diuresis, clears heat

Conditions: food retention, stomach heat, swelling, arthritis, spasms

Folk Remedies:
1. HYPERTENSION - boil tea for 4 hours; drink lukewarm, daily over a period of 1 month.

2. WARTS - eat only steamed soybean sprouts for 3 days consecutively without anything else.

SPINACH

Nature / Taste: cool and sweet

Actions: strengthens all organs, lubricates intestines, promotes urination, ventilates the chest, quenches thirst

Conditions: constipation, thirst, tightness in chest, inability to urinate, night blindness, alcohol intoxication, diabetes

Contraindications: Not to be used with diarrhea, or a history of kidney stones. Also, spinach does not mix well with tofu or dairy products due to the unhealthy combination that results from the oxalic acid in the spinach and the high calcium foods. This can lead to crystallized stones in the kidneys, if one is so predisposed.

Folk Remedies:

1. ACUTE CONJUNCTIVITIS - simmer spinach and chrysanthemum flowers; drink the liquid.

2. NIGHT BLINDNESS - fresh spinach juice, drink 1 cup 2 times daily.

3. DIABETES - boil tea from spinach and chicken gizzard, drink 1 cup 3 times daily.

4. CONSTIPATION, URINARY OBSTRUCTION, HEADACHE - drink spinach soup.

SQUASH (SUMMER SQUASH, ZUCCHINI)

SUMMER SQUASH includes all the soft skin varieties. See PUMPKIN for properties of WINTER SQUASH.

Nature / Taste: cool and sweet

Actions: clears heat, detoxifies, promotes diuresis, quenches thirst, relieves restlessness

Conditions: skin lesions, difficulty urinating, edema, summer heat, irritability, thirst

Contraindications: Not to be used in beriberi or scabies.

Folk Remedies:
1. BURNS - preserve cut up squash until it becomes liquid (usually 6 - 12 months) and apply the liquid to the burn.

2. EDEMA IN THE EXTREMITIES OR THE AB-DOMEN - cook squash with vinegar until soggy and eat on empty stomach or make tea from squash skin.

3. SUMMER HEAT AND IRRITABILITY - eat squash as a salad.

4. JAUNDICE - drink tea made from squash skin, 1 cup 3 times daily.

SWEET POTATO (YAM)

Nature / Taste: neutral and sweet

Actions: strengthens spleen and stomach function, tonifies Chi, clears heat, detoxifies, increases the production of milk

Conditions: bloody stools, diarrhea, constipation, jaundice, edema, ascites, night blindness, diabetes, breast abscess, boils, skin lesions

Contraindications: Overeating sweet potatoes will cause gas, heartburn, indigestion, abdominal distention and acid regurgitation.

Folk Remedies:
1. NIGHT BLINDNESS - cook yam or sweet potato with animal liver (preferably goat).

2. JAUNDICE - cook yam soup with squash and pearl barley.

3. SHINGLES AND BREAST ABSCESS - apply grated, raw yam locally or mix in a pinch of borax.

4. ECZEMA (PARTICULARLY GENITAL ECZEMA) - make tea with sweet potato and a pinch of salt and bathe the area. Sprinkle afterwards with natural talcum powder.

5. POISON INSECT BITES - mash yam or sweet potato with honey and apply.

6. CIRRHOSIS OF THE LIVER AND ACCOMPANY-ING EDEMA IN THE ABDOMEN - apply to the navel a mixture of mashed sweet potato and brown sugar; change hourly.

7. DIABETES - cook soup with winter melon.

8. BLOODY STOOLS - mix sweet potato powder or yam powder with honey.

TARO ROOT

Nature / Taste: neutral, sweet and pungent

Actions: clears heat, reduces swelling, benefits spleen, regulates digestive system

Conditions: swollen lymph glands, nodules, goiters, externally for pain from tendinitis, sprains, traumas, snake bites, bee stings

Contraindications: If you eat too much, it can cause food retention and stomach pains. Externally, can cause allergic reaction in some people; an antidote for this would be to apply fresh ginger juice. Also, taro root is slightly toxic raw.

Folk Remedies:

1. EXTERNALLY FOR INFECTIONS SUCH AS PLEURISY, PERITONITIS, APPENDICITIS, JOINT PAIN, SCIATICA, BACK PAIN, ARTHRITIS - mix together peeled taro root and ginger, mixed into a paste with some flour and water, and apply to the affected area. Cover

with a cloth. During the winter time, heat up the paste and apply. Change daily and always apply fresh.

2. SNAKE BITE, BEE STING, AND BUG BITES - mash taro root with a pinch of salt and apply locally.

3 BLISTERS THAT CONTAIN FLUID - charcoal taro to ash, mix with sesame oil and apply to blister.

4. SWOLLEN LYMPH GLANDS, NODULES, SCROFULA, GOITER, AND T.B. - dry taro root, grind to powder, then take equal parts of water chestnuts and jelly fish and boil into tea. Take the liquid and mix with the taro root powder; roll into pills the size of mung beans, take 2 T. of pills 3 times daily with warm water.

TURNIP

Nature / Taste: cool, sweet, bitter and pungent

Actions: clears heat, removes dampness, removes stagnant food, detoxifies, stops cough

Conditions: boils, breast abscesses, diabetes, tinea (ringworm), baldness in children

Folk Remedies:
1. ABSCESSES - apply grated raw turnip bulbs mixed with a tablespoon of salt.

2. BALDING IN CHILDREN - charcoal turnip greens and mix with sesame oil; apply to bald spots.

WATER CHESTNUT

Nature / Taste: cold and sweet

Actions: clears heat and stops bleeding

Conditions: dry cough due to heat in the lung with thick, tenacious mucus, jaundice, bloody stool, excessive uterine bleeding, antidote for lead and copper poisoning

Folk Remedies

1. BLOODY STOOLS - juice fresh water chestnuts and mix with equal amount of rice wine and drink 3 times a day on an empty stomach. Results should be seen within 3 days.

2. EXCESS UTERINE BLEEDING - charcoal the water chestnuts, powder them and take with rice wine.

3. BRONCHITIS, PNEUMONIA, COUGH - make tea from fresh water chestnuts and honeysuckle flowers; drink 3 - 5 cups per day.

4. LEAD AND COPPER POISONING - consume daily 1 pound of fresh water chestnuts with 1/4 pound of peach kernels.

WATERCRESS

Nature / Taste: cool and bitter

Actions: clears heat, quenches thirst, lubricates lungs, promotes diuresis

Conditions: thirst, irritability, restlessness, sore and dry throat, cough with yellow sputum

Contraindications: Not to be used case of in diarrhea.

Folk Remedies:

1. THIRST, IRRITABILITY, AND SORE THROAT - drink fresh raw watercress juice.

2. COUGH - boil tea from watercress and apricot kernels (or almonds). Remove the apex of the apricot kernel which is toxic. Drink 1 cup 3 times daily.

WINTER MELON

Nature / Taste: cool, sweet and bland

Actions: clears heat, detoxifies, promotes urination, quenches thirst, relieves irritability, dispels dampness, antidote for seafood poisoning

Conditions: boils, skin lesions, ascites (edema in the abdomen), difficult urination, heatstroke

Folk Remedies:

1. HIVES - make tea of winter melon skin and drink.

2. CHRONIC NEPHRITIS - cook winter melon with poi and no salt.

3. DIFFICULTY URINATING - drink the fresh juice with honey.

4. HEATSTROKE - make winter melon soup and drink 3 times daily.

5. PROMOTE LACTATION - cook winter melon rind with trout.

6. SUMMER HEAT WITH CONTINUOUS HIGH FEVER - make tea from winter melon rind and grapefruit seeds (remove shells or crush seeds) and drink constantly.

FRUITS

APPLE

Nature / Taste: cool, sweet and slightly sour

Actions: strengthens heart, tonifies Chi, quenches thirst, promotes body fluids, lubricates lungs, resolves mucus

Conditions: dry throat, dehydration, indigestion, hypertension, constipation, chronic diarrhea

Folk Remedies:

1. CONSTIPATION - eat a fresh apple on an empty stomach.

2. INDIGESTION - eat an apple after each meal.

3. DIARRHEA - take 2 teaspoons of powdered, dried apple 3 times daily on an empty stomach.

4. COUGH WITH YELLOW SPUTUM - drink apple juice.

5. HYPERTENSION - eat 3 apples a day.

6. GENERAL CLEANSING - fast one day a week on apples, apple juice, and beet top tea. The apples contain pectin which acts as a broom in our intestines.

For problems of a cold nature, bake the apples to decrease their cooling properties.

APRICOT

Nature / Taste: slightly cool, sweet and sour

Actions: regenerates body fluids, clears heat, detoxifies, quenches thirst

Conditions: dehydration, thirst, cough

Contraindications: Too much injures bones and tendons and produces mucus; in children this can cause skin rashes. Not good to eat too many during pregnancy.

Folk Remedies:
1. SUMMER THIRST AND DEHYDRATION - eat fresh apricots (no more than 5-10).
2. COUGH - make tea from 1 teaspoon of ground apricot kernels, adding a bit of honey. The inner kernel of the apricot seed is used to ventilate lungs, descend rebellious Chi, lubricate intestines, relieve constipation, relieve cough and asthma. One should remove the apex of the kernel which is toxic.

BANANA

Nature / Taste: cold and sweet

Actions: clears heat, lubricates lungs, lubricates intestines, lowers blood pressure, aids alcohol intoxication

Conditions: constipation, thirst, cough, hemorrhoids, hypertension, alcohol intoxication

Contraindications: Not to be used in cold conditions.

Folk Remedies:
1. HEMORRHOIDS AND CONSTIPATION - eat a banana every day on an empty stomach.

2. HYPERTENSION - drink banana peel (organic) tea.

3. COUGH - cook banana with a bit of sugar. Note, this may not be appropriate for Americans who already consume about 120 pounds of sugar a year. If honey is substituted, do not cook the honey.

CANTALOUPE

Nature / Taste: cold and sweet

Actions: clears heat, quenches thirst, relieves summer heat problems, eases urination

Conditions: summer heat thirst, lung abscess, irritability

Contraindications: Not for cold conditions, history of coughing or vomiting blood, diarrhea, ulcers, heart disease, or weak stomach. Melons rot easily in the stomach and thus should be eaten alone.

Folk Remedies:

1. TO INDUCE VOMITING - take dried, ground cantaloupe seeds in warm water.

CHERRY

Nature / Taste: warm and sweet

Actions: benefits skin and overall body, rejuvenates, strengthens spleen, stimulates appetite, stops dysentery and diarrhea, quenches thirst, regenerates fluids, stops seminal emissions, prolongs life

Conditions: measles, burns, diarrhea, dysentery, thirst, premature ejaculation

Contraindications: Eaten in excess will cause nausea, vomiting, skin lesions and cause a person to feel hot. This injures the bones and tendons.

Folk Remedies:

1. MEASLES - drink fresh warmed cherry juice.

2. BURNS - apply locally.

3. ENLARGED THYROID OR GOITER - soak cherry pits in vinegar until they disintegrate, then apply locally.

4. HERNIA PAIN - fry cherry pits with vinegar, mash to powder; take 1 teaspoon per dose.

CHINESE DATE (RED OR BLACK JUJUBE)

Nature / Taste: neutral* and sweet

Actions: strengthens spleen, tonifies Yin, nourishes the body, tonifies blood, lubricates lungs, stops coughs, stops diarrhea, harmonizes within the body or within an herb formula (dates and licorice can reduce the harshness of a food or herb and unite the combination into action).

Conditions: Yin deficiency, weak digestion, cough, night sweats, weakness, anemia, blood in urine, diarrhea, bruises, nervous hysteria

Contraindications: Too much creates mucus, distended stomach, and is hard on the teeth.

Folk Remedies:

1. BLOOD IN URINE - drink red date tea.

2. SPONTANEOUS SWEATING - boil tea from 10 red dates and 10 preserved plums.

The black dates are slightly warming.

CHINESE PRUNE

These prunes are made from half ripened plums and have a sour flavor. They are more beneficial therapeutically than the sweet variety that is made from fully ripened plums.

Nature / Taste: warm and sour

Actions: astringes intestines, stops diarrhea, kills worms, stops cough, consolidates the lungs, quenches thirst, promotes body fluids. The sweet prunes quench thirst, promote body fluids, and moisten the intestines.

Folk Remedies:

1. DYSENTERY - for both prevention (as before a trip to India or Mexico) and treatment, brew prune tea and take before meals on empty stomach.

2. INTESTINAL WORMS - make tea with prunes and black pepper.

3. FISH BONES STUCK IN THE THROAT - brew concentrated prune tea and add an equal part of rice vinegar; drink slowly. The herb clematis, powdered and mixed with rice vinegar could be given in an emergency, to dissolve a fish bone.

4. SUMMER HEAT IRRITABILITY - drink prune juice.

COCONUT

Nature / Taste: warm and sweet

Actions: strengthens the body, reduces swelling, stops bleeding, kills worms, activates heart function

Conditions: weakness, nosebleeds, intestinal or skin worms

Folk Remedies:

1. WORMS - every morning on an empty stomach, drink the juice and eat the meat of 1/2 coconut; wait 3 hours before eating anything else.

2. EDEMA DUE TO WEAK HEART - drink plenty of coconut juice.

The milk inside of the coconut is neutral and sweet

FIG

Nature / Taste: cool and sweet

Actions: clears heat, lubricates lungs and intestines, stops diarrhea

Conditions: dry cough, dry throat, lung heat, constipation, indigestion, hemorrhoids, prolapse of the rectum

Folk Remedies:
1. LUNG HEAT SYMPTOMS - make tea from figs (preferably fresh).
2. HEMORRHOIDS - bathe area in fig tea.
3. ASTHMA - blend fig juice and drink 3 times daily.
4. HERNIA - drink fig and fennel tea.

GRAPE

Nature / Taste: warm, sweet and sour

Actions: very tonifying (particularly the red or purple varieties), nourishes blood, strengthens bones and tendons, tonifies Chi, harmonizes stomach, promotes diuresis, relieves irritability

Conditions: cold type arthritis, tendinitis, painful urination, hepatitis, jaundice, anemia, flu

Contraindications: Grape wine should not be combined with fatty foods because it can result in phlegm and heat that rises to the heart and can cause strokes and heart attacks. Also, excessive consumption of grapes leads to constipation or diarrhea.

Folk Remedies:
1. ANEMIA - eat raisins.

2. ARTHRITIS (COLD TYPE) AND TENDINITIS - make grape vine tea and add some grape wine. The moderate use of grape wine can be of benefit in cold environments and cold conditions.

3. HEPATITIS AND JAUNDICE - make grape tea.

4. FLU - drink grape juice.

GRAPEFRUIT

Nature / Taste: cold, sweet and sour

Actions: strengthens stomach, aids digestion, circulates Chi, detoxifies alcohol intoxication

Conditions: decreased appetite, weak digestion, stomach fullness, alcohol intoxication, dry cough

Folk Remedies:

1. DRY COUGH - cook 4 grapefruit slices with either pork or cabbage.

2. CHRONIC COUGH - make tea from about 20 grapefruit seeds, adding a bit of honey; drink 3 times daily.

3. JAUNDICE AND STOMACH DISTENTION - char and powder grapefruit peel*; take a teaspoon with warm water 3 times daily.

4. GASTRITIS OR INFLAMMATION OF THE STOMACH - make tea from aged grapefruit peel, green tea leaves, and 2 slices of fresh ginger; drink all day.

5. FROSTBITE - wash or soak area in grapefruit peel tea.

*GRAPEFRUIT PEEL is warming and can be used to dispel cold, regulate Chi, aid digestion, dry dampness, resolve sputum, aid wind-cold cough, stomach distention and scratchy throat. Make tea from the dried peel.

HAWTHORN BERRY

Nature / Taste: slightly warm, sweet and sour

Actions: strengthens spleen, removes stagnant food, invigorates blood, dissolves sputum, relieves stagnant Chi, aids digestion

Conditions: food stagnation (especially meat), bloody stools, abdominal pain, absence of menstruation due to blood stagnation, poor appetite, hypertension, high cholesterol

Folk Remedies:
1. CHILD WITH NO APPETITE - give the berries or tea daily.

2. HYPERTENSION - drink tea daily.

LEMON

Nature / Taste: cool and sour

Actions: regenerates body fluids, harmonizes stomach, regulates Chi, quenches thirst, benefits liver

Conditions: sore throat, dry mouth, stomach distention, cough

Folk Remedies:
1. HYPERTENSION - make tea from 1 peeled lemon, 10 fresh water chestnuts, and 2 1/2 cups of water; drink once daily.

2. SORE THROAT - drink lemon tea with honey.

3. REGULATE CHI, BENEFIT LIVER - squeeze 1/2 lemon in warm water and drink every morning.

LITCHI FRUIT (LYCHEE)

Nature / Taste: warm, sweet and astringent

Actions: nourishes blood, calms spirit, soothes liver, regulates Chi

Conditions: hernia, weak and deficient conditions, irritability, restless heart

Contraindications: Over consumption can lead to nosebleed, feverish sensation, thirst, and can induce the onset of smallpox or chicken pox. Not to be used in any type of heat condition.

Folk Remedies:

1. WEAK CONDITIONS, BLOOD DEFICIENCY - take dried litchi and black jujube date and boil tea (7 of each); drink daily.

2. BED-WETTING - eat 10 dried litchis daily.

3. NAUSEA, VOMITING, BURPING, AND BELCHING - take dried litchi with the kernel, charcoal, powder and take with warm water.

4. BLEEDING AFTER BIRTH OR ABORTION - take 7 dried litchis, mash and boil with 2 cups of water; reduce to 1 cup, drink 3 times daily until the bleeding stops.

5. HERNIA - take litchi kernel, bake and grind to powder; take 1 teaspoon on an empty stomach daily. Or, grind the litchi kernel, mix with rice wine and take every morning on an empty stomach.

LOQUAT

Nature / Taste: neutral, sweet and sour

Actions: lubricates dryness, stops cough, harmonizes stomach, descends rebellious Chi, calms the liver

Conditions: dry mouth, thirst, irritability, dry cough, nausea, vomiting

Folk Remedies:
1. VOMITING AND NAUSEA - boil tea.
2. COUGH - eat fresh.

MANGO

Nature / Taste: neutral, sweet and sour

Actions: regenerates body fluids, stops cough, stops thirst, strengthens stomach

Conditions: cough, thirst, poor digestion, enlarged prostate, nausea

Contraindication: overeating can cause itching or skin eruptions

Folk Remedies:
1. ENLARGED PROSTATE - boil mango peel and seed into tea.
2. WEAK DIGESTION - drink mango juice.

MULBERRY

Nature / Taste: slightly cold and sweet

Actions: quenches thirst, detoxifies, nourishes blood, tonifies kidneys, lubricates lungs, relieves constipation, calms the spirit, promotes diuresis

Conditions: thirst, irritability, dry mouth, diabetes, anemia, constipation, back pain due to kidney weakness, alcohol intoxication, lymph node enlargement, blurred vision

Folk Remedies:

1. COUGH - take 2 teaspoons 2 times daily of mulberry syrup, made by cooking mulberries on low flame until they dissolve, then adding honey and cooking down to a thick syrup.

2. CONSTIPATION - drink mulberry juice.

3. INSOMNIA - boil mulberry tea and take 1/2 cup.

ORANGE

Nature / Taste: cool, sweet and sour

Actions: lubricates lungs, resolves mucus, increases appetite, strengthens spleen, quenches thirst, promotes body fluids

Conditions: thirst, dehydration, stagnant Chi, hernia

Folk Remedies:

1. COUGH WITH LOTS OF MUCUS - cook the orange and eat it.

2. STUCK MUCUS, STAGNANT CHI, CHEST FULLNESS OR DISTENTION - make tea from unsprayed, dried orange peel.*

3. CHI STAGNATION, PROSTATE ENLARGEMENT AND HERNIA - make tea from orange seeds.

ORANGE PEEL is warm, bitter and pungent, and is used to invigorate the movement of Chi and dry dampness.

PAPAYA

Nature / Taste: neutral, sweet and sour

Actions: strengthens stomach and spleen, aids digestion, clears summer heat, lubricates lungs, stops cough, aids irritability, kills worms, increases milk production

Conditions: cough, indigestion, stomachache, eczema, skin lesions, intestinal worms

Folk Remedies:

1. INCREASING MILK PRODUCTION - put fresh papaya in fish soup.

2. COUGH - peel and steam papaya, then add honey.

3. STOMACHACHE AND INDIGESTION - cook papaya and eat with or after meals.

4. INTESTINAL WORMS - sun dry green papaya, powder, and take 2 teaspoons on an empty stomach every morning.

5. SKIN LESIONS - apply fresh papaya.

DRIED PAPAYA is warm, sweet and sour. It is used to invigorate and activate the channels, aid digestion, and resolve dampness.

PEACH

Nature / Taste: very cool, sweet and slightly sour

Actions: lubricates lungs, clears heat, aids diabetes, promotes body fluids, induces sweating

Conditions: diabetes, dry cough, intestinal worms, vaginitis

Contraindications: Not to be used with damp and cold conditions.

Folk Remedies:

1. INDUCING SWEATING OR KILLING WORMS - drink peach leaf tea.

2. PROMOTING BLOOD CIRCULATION - make tea from the innermost seed, the kernel.

3. DRY COUGH - eat fresh peaches.

4. VAGINITIS - douche with peach leaf tea.

PEAR APPLE (ASIAN PEAR)

Nature / Taste: cold and sweet

Actions: regenerates body fluids, quenches thirst, calms the heart, lubricates lungs, relieves restlessness, promotes urination, clears heat, detoxifies, lubricates the throat, dissolves mucus, descends Chi and stops cough

Conditions: cough due to heat in the lungs, excess mucus, irritability, thirst, dry throat, hoarse throat, retina pain, constipation, difficult urination, skin lesions, alcohol intoxication

Contraindications: Not to be used with cold stomach and spleen, manifesting as cold extremities or diarrhea. Also, not to be used by pregnant women, or in cases of anemia.

Folk Remedies:

1. COUGH AND BRONCHITIS - core the pear and steam it; eat 3-4 times daily. Pear can also be cooked with scallions.

2. COUGH WITH YELLOW PHLEGM - core pear, and fill with 3 grams powdered fritillaria bulb (Chuan Bei Mu) and a little rock sugar or brown sugar; steam about 30 minutes and eat the whole thing.

3. ACUTE VOICE LOSS - peel and juice 2-3 pears, adding 2 teaspoons of honey.

4. WHOOPING COUGH - core the pear and insert 1/2 gram of ephedra; steam, then remove the herb and eat the pear.

5. NAUSEA, BELCHING - core the pear and insert 10-15 cloves; steam, then remove the cloves and eat the pear.

6. ALCOHOL INTOXICATION - drink pear juice or tea to prevent hangover.

DOMESTIC PEAR has the same properties as the ASIAN PEAR, but it is milder.

PERSIMMON

Nature: / Taste: cool, sweet and astringent

Actions: lubricates lungs, stops cough with heat, dissolves sputum, strengthens spleen, stops diarrhea, quenches thirst, clears heat

Conditions: pain in the throat due to heat, cough, thirst, vomiting blood, dysentery, alcohol intoxication

Contraindications: Do not eat persimmons along with crabs as the combination produces extreme diarrhea.

Folk Remedies:

1. VOMITING OR COUGHING BLOOD - cook a partially ripened persimmon in rice wine for 10 minutes; eat the persimmon. Another remedy is to take dried, charred persimmon powder in warm water.

2. BLEEDING ULCERS AND LOWER INTESTINAL BLEEDING - take dried, charred, powdered persimmon in warm water (about a tablespoon of the powder).

3. HYPERTENSION - drink 3 glasses daily of unripened persimmon juice.

4. NAUSEA AND VOMITING - add dried persimmon to water to make a mush, steam it and take 2 tablespoons 3 times daily for 3-4 days or until condition ceases. Cloves could be a good addition; or make persimmon *cap* and cloves tea.

5. ALCOHOL INTOXICATION - take persimmon juice or tea.

6. ULCERATED SKIN LESIONS - apply a combination of charred persimmon powder and black pepper.

PINEAPPLE

Nature / Taste: warm, sweet and sour

Actions: aids digestion, stops diarrhea, dispels summer heat

Conditions: heat stroke, irritability, thirst, indigestion, diarrhea

Contraindications: Pineapples are slightly toxic; this can be neutralized by washing with salt water. Pineapple is also said to generate dampness, so not to be used in those situations.

Folk Remedies:
1. HEAT STROKE AND IRRITABILITY - drink fresh juice.

2. NEPHRITIS (KIDNEY INFLAMMATION) - make tea from peeled pineapple and reed roots; drink freely throughout the day.

3. BRONCHITIS - boil tea and add honey.

4. DYSENTERY - boil tea.

PLUM

Nature / Taste: slightly warm, sweet and sour

Actions: stimulates appetite, aids digestion, regulates body fluids, stops thirst, softens or soothes the liver, removes stagnation of Chi, removes the feeling of *steaming bones*

Conditions: dehydration, thirst, Chi stagnation, erratic energy flow, poor digestion, dysentery

Contraindications: Too many plums are not good for the teeth.

Folk Remedies:
1. DYSENTERY - drink plum skin tea.

RASPBERRY

Nature / Taste: slightly warm, sweet and sour

Actions: tonifies liver and kidneys, astringes essence, astringes urination, brightens the eyes

Conditions: kidney and liver deficiency, blurry vision, spermatorrhea, seminal emission, frequent urination

Folk Remedies:
1. IMPOTENCE AND SEMINAL EMISSION - take dry raspberries, charcoal and grind to powder; take 3 teaspoons every night before bed with some rice wine.

2. BED-WETTING OR FREQUENT URINATION - take charcoaled raspberry powder, make tea and drink before bedtime every night.

3. ECZEMA, SKIN LESIONS, AND FUNGUS CONDITIONS - boil fresh raspberries to a concentrate; wash area with this.

RASPBERRY LEAF is very strengthening to the female system, and can be used throughout pregnancy, as well as other phases of the woman's life. It is generally taken as tea.

STRAWBERRY

Nature / Taste: cool, sweet and sour

Actions: lubricates lungs, promotes body fluids, strengthens spleen, detoxifies in alcohol intoxication

Conditions: dry cough, sore throat, difficult urination, food retention, lack of appetite

Folk Remedies:
1. DRY COUGH - mash strawberries with brown sugar; steam and eat 3 times daily.

2. DRY THROAT, THIRST, HOARSE VOICE, SORE THROAT - take 1 glass fresh strawberry juice 2 times daily.

3. DIFFICULT URINATION - mash fresh strawberries, add cold water; drink 3 times daily.

4. LACK OF APPETITE, FOOD RETENTION, ABDOMINAL DISTENTION AND PAIN - eat 5 strawberries before each meal.

TANGERINE

Nature / Taste: warm, sweet and sour

Actions: carminative, opens the channels, strengthens the stomach, stops cough

Conditions: nausea, vomiting, cough, excess white or clear mucus, chest tightness, rib pain

Folk Remedies:
1. NAUSEA, VOMITING, STOMACH DISCOMFORT -

make tea from unsprayed tangerine peels*, fresh ginger root and cardamon seeds.

2. CHEST FULLNESS, PAIN IN RIBS - use tangerine fruit combined with rice wine and water to make a tea.

3. HERNIA, TESTICULAR PAIN - roast equal parts of tangerine seeds and fennel seeds; grind to powder. Take 3 - 6 grams with warm sake before bed.

*TANGERINE PEEL is warm, pungent and bitter; carminative, arrests cough, strengthens the stomach and resolves phlegm.

TOMATO

Nature / Taste: slightly cool, sweet and sour

Actions: promotes body fluids, quenches thirst, strengthens stomach, aids digestion, cools blood, clears heat, detoxifies, calms the liver, removes stagnant food

Conditions: liver heat rising, hypertension, bloodshot eyes, dehydration, indigestion due to low stomach acid, food retention, kidney infection

Folk Remedies:
1. HYPERTENSION AND EYE HEMORRHAGE - take 2 raw tomatoes on an empty stomach, every day for 1 month; also avoid spicy foods.

2. KIDNEY DISEASE - eat at least 1 raw tomato per day.

3. INDIGESTION AND FOOD RETENTION - eat 1/2 - 1 fresh tomato after meals.

WATERMELON

Nature / Taste: cold and sweet

Actions: quenches thirst, relieves irritability, dispels summer heat problems, promotes diuresis, detoxifies

Conditions: sores, dry mouth, summer heat irritability, bloody dysentery, jaundice, edema, difficult urination

Contraindications: Not to be used in cold conditions, with weak stomach, or with polyuria.

Folk Remedies:

1. EDEMA FROM NEPHRITIS - boil tea from the rind and the inner portion.

2. JAUNDICE - boil tea from the rind and red beans.

3. FLUID IN THE ABDOMEN - make tea from the skins of watermelon, squash, and winter melon.

4. CONSTIPATION - boil tea from watermelon seeds or grind into meal and take with warm water.

GRAINS

BUCKWHEAT

Nature / Taste: neutral and sweet

Actions: descends Chi, strengthens stomach, stops dysentery, lowers blood pressure, strengthens blood vessels

Conditions: chronic diarrhea, dysentery, spontaneous sweating, hypertension, skin lesions

Folk Remedies:

1. SKIN LESIONS - boil tea and wash area. Or, roast buckwheat, grind to powder and mix with rice vinegar to make a paste; then apply to area.

2. LEUKORRHEA AND CHRONIC DIARRHEA - grind roasted buckwheat, mix with warm water and take 2 teaspoons 2 times daily.

3. HIGH BLOOD PRESSURE - make tea from buckwheat and lotus roots.

4. HEMORRHOIDS - mix rooster bile with buckwheat meal and roll in pill form. Take 1 t. twice daily.

CORN MEAL

Nature / Taste: neutral and sweet

Actions: tonify Chi, strengthen the stomach and spleen, benefit the heart, diuretic, stimulate the flow of bile

Conditions: weak digestion, heart disease, high blood pressure, edema, gallstones

Folk Remedies:

1. WEAK DIGESTION - make a soupy porridge with corn

meal. This is an easy to digest meal for recovery from a flu or cold.

2. EDEMA, DIFFICULT URINATION, HYPERTEN-SION - eat corn meal regularly and drink corn silk tea.

FRESH CORN and CORN SILK are cooling and more diuretic than the dried CORN MEAL.

MILLET

Nature / Taste: cool and sweet

Actions: stops vomiting, relieves diarrhea, consolidates or astringes the stomach and intestines, clears heat, promotes urination, soothes morning sickness

Folk Remedies:

1. MORNING SICKNESS AND VOMITING - eat millet porridge as a regular staple; may add fresh ginger.

2. DIARRHEA - roast millet until aromatic; eat 1/2 cup 3 times daily.

3. OBSTRUCTED URINATION - boil tea from millet and add 1/2 teaspoon brown sugar.

4. DIABETES - steam millet with yams and jujube dates.

OATS

Nature / Taste: warm and sweet

Actions: strengthens spleen, tonifies Chi, harmonizes stomach, regulates Chi, carminative, stops lactation (sprouted form only)

Conditions: lack of appetite, indigestion, abdominal distention and fullness, dysentery, swelling

Folk Remedies:

1. STOP LACTATION - boil sprouted oats or sprouted barley tea and drink 1 cup 3 times daily, or use barley malt as a sweetener in the diet.

2. SWELLING - cook oats and azuki or mung beans to a mush.

3. POSTPARTUM URINARY AND BOWEL OBSTRUCTION - roast sprouted oats, grind into meal, take 2 t. 3 times a day with lukewarm water.

4. HEPATITIS - make tea from sprouted oats and dried orange peels, drink 1 c. 3 times daily.

PEARL BARLEY (COIX, JOB'S TEARS)

Nature / Taste: cool and bland

Actions: promotes diuresis, strengthens spleen, benefits gall bladder, clears heat, detoxifies

Conditions: swelling, indigestion, diarrhea, jaundice, tumors, dysuria

Folk Remedies:

1. FOR QUITTING COFFEE - substitute roasted barley tea for the coffee.

2. SWELLING - eat pearl barley soup.

3. HEAT AND DAMP CONDITIONS - make a soupy porridge of mung beans and pearl barley and eat daily.

4. HEAT CONDITIONS AND SKIN LESIONS - blend barley and water, boil, and drink the liquid.

5. SKIN LESIONS WITH PUS DISCHARGE - sprinkle pearl barley powder locally.

6. ACNE - mix pearl barley powder with aloe vera gel and make a facial mask to be applied every night before bed. Leave on overnight and wash off with water in the morning.

PEARLED BARLEY, the common one here in the supermarkets, is smaller and milder than this Chinese herb variety. They can be used interchangeably. COIX has a stronger taste and is more diuretic.

RICE (BROWN)

Nature / Taste: neutral and sweet

Actions: strengthens spleen, nourishes stomach, quenches thirst, relieves irritability, astringes intestines, stops diarrhea

Conditions: indigestion, diarrhea, vomiting, nausea, summer heat irritability

Folk Remedies:
1. BLOODY DYSENTERY - cook brown rice with the persimmon *cap;* eat the rice.

2. DIGESTIVE AID - eat fermented rice cake after each meal.

3. CHILD REGURGITATING MOTHER'S MILK - roast rice until overdone (brownish-black), add water and cook; give the child the fluid.

4. DIARRHEA - grind rice, charcoal and take 1 - 2 teaspoons each time, 3 times daily.

5. ANOREXIA AND DIGESTIVE WEAKNESS - 1/2 c. over-done rice (bottom of pot) mixed with cardamon, fennel and orange peel, and cooked into porridge.

6. DIFFICULTLY URINATING - consume rice porridge continuously for one month.

RICE (SWEET)

Nature / Taste: warm and sweet

Actions: warms spleen and stomach, tonifies Chi, astringes urine

Conditions: stomach pains due to cold, diabetes, frequent urination, obesity, anemia

Contraindications: Eating too much will cause indigestion.

Folk Remedies:
1. OBESITY - eat sweet rice cake (mochi); a small amount is very filling.

2. INDIGESTION - make tea from malt and sweet rice sprouts.

3. ANEMIA, LUNG TUBERCULOSIS - cook sweet rice porridge with red dates and pearl barley and eat regularly.

4. SPONTANEOUS SWEATING - dry roast sweet rice and wheat bran, grind into meal; take 1 tablespoon 3 times daily.

5. STOMACH PAINS DUE TO COLD, DIARRHEA - make sweet rice porridge with yams, lotus seeds, Chinese red dates, and a pinch of pepper.

RICE (WHITE)

Nature / Taste: slightly cool and sweet

Actions: moistens Yin, clears heat, diuretic, reduces swelling

Conditions: febrile diseases, swelling, vomiting of blood, nosebleeds, nausea

Folk Remedies:
1. CHRONIC GASTRITIS - burn rice, powder it and take twice daily with ginger tea before meals for 3 consecutive

days, followed by a liquid diet, avoiding cold, raw and oily foods.

2. VOMITING DUE TO FEBRILE DISEASE - consume rice porridge.

3. FOOD RETENTION - wash rice thoroughly, then bring rice to a boil, add aloe vera juice and drink the liquid. This will produce a loose stool and reduction of the stomach distress.

RICE BRAN

Nature / Taste: neutral and sweet

Actions: dispels dampness, diuretic

Conditions: mild edema in legs and feet, high cholesterol

Folk Remedies
1. HIGH CHOLESTEROL - add rice bran to a grain dish every day for at least 2 months

RYE

Nature / Taste: neutral and sweet

Actions: arrests perspiration due to weakness, strengthens Stomach, fortifies Chi

Conditions: fatigue, lethargy, night or day sweats due to weakness, fetal retention (baby has died, but not yet expelled by mother)

Folk Remedies:
1. WEAKNESS TYPE PERSPIRATION - boil whole rye for 15-20 minutes, add molasses and drink the liquid.

2. FETAL RETENTION - make tea from the entire rye plant and raspberry leaves, and drink as much as possible.

WHEAT

Nature / Taste: slightly cool and sweet

Actions: clears heat, quenches thirst, relieves restlessness, promotes diuresis, calms spirit, stops sweating

Conditions: dry mouth and throat, swelling, difficult urination, insomnia, irritability, restlessness, menopause, spontaneous sweating, night sweats, diarrhea, burns

Contraindications: Always use organically grown wheat. Wheat absorbs 10 times more nitrates (like from chemical fertilizers) than any other grain. This could explain the high incidence of allergies to modern day wheat.

Folk Remedies:

1. INSOMNIA, MENOPAUSE, RESTLESSNESS - make tea from 1 c. wheat, 12 grams licorice, and 15 Chinese black dates. Drink 1 c. 3 times daily.

2. BURNS (INITIAL STAGES) - make a paste of charcoaled wheat meal and sesame oil and apply locally.

3. SWELLING, DIFFICULT URINATION - make tea from wheat and pearl barley.

4. SPONTANEOUS SWEATING - make tea from wheat, crushed oyster shells and Chinese red dates.

WHEAT BRAN

Nature / Taste: slightly warm, sweet

Actions: calms the spirit, resolves dampness, moves stool

Conditions: agitation, swelling, high cholesterol, constipation

Contraindications: Not for use in colitis; can be irritating.

Folk Remedies

1. RESTLESSNESS AND EMOTIONAL INSTABILITY -
make a tea of wheat bran, licorice root and Chinese jujube
dates. Drink 3 times a day until symptoms are relieved.

2. CONSTIPATION - add wheat bran to diet regularly, being
sure to drink plenty of water too. Psyllium seed products will
also provide excellent bulk laxative action.

WHEAT GERM

Nature / Taste: warm and sweet

Actions: relieves restlessness, arrests diabetes

Conditions: emotional agitation, diabetes

Contraindications: Always buy wheat germ fresh, and store
in the refrigerator. Due to the high oil content of wheat germ
it can go rancid if not properly stored. Rancid oil will cause
a burning sensation in the throat.

Folk Remedies

1. DIABETES - make bread from 60% wheat germ and 40%
whole wheat flour with an egg added in. Ideally, consume up
to 1.5 pounds of wheat germ per day.

SEEDS, NUTS & LEGUMES

ALMOND

Nature / Taste: neutral and sweet

Actions: ventilates lungs, relieves cough and asthma, transform phlegm, lubricates intestines

Conditions: lung conditions, asthma, constipation, cough

Folk Remedies:
1. COUGH AND ASTHMA - grind almonds to a fine meal, add fructose; dissolve 2 tablespoons in water.

AZUKI BEAN (ADUKI, RED)

Nature / Taste: neutral, sweet and sour

Actions: strengthens spleen, benefits diabetes, counteracts toxins, reduces dampness, benefits kidneys

Conditions: mumps, diabetes, leukorrhea, excessive thirst, hunger, or excretion of fluids, edema

Folk Remedies:
1. DIABETES - after soaking red beans, boil 2 hours, drink the liquid 3 times daily.

2. MUMPS - mash sprouted red beans and apply, either alone or mixed with dandelion.

BLACK BEAN

Nature / Taste: warm and sweet

Actions: tonifies kidneys, nourishes the Yin, strengthens and nourishes blood, brightens eyes, promotes diuresis, and strengthens kidneys

Conditions: lower back pain, knee pain, infertility, seminal emissions, blurry vision, ear problems, difficult urination

Folk Remedies:

1. BERIBERI - cook black beans with carp.

2. SPONTANEOUS MENOPAUSAL SWEATING - make boiled black bean juice.

3. LOW BACK PAIN, WEAK KNEES, FREQUENT URINATION, AND OTHER KIDNEY WEAKNESS SYMPTOMS - slowly cook (for about 2-3 hours) 1/2 cup black beans, 1/2 cup water, and 3/4 cup rice wine. This is a good winter tonic.

4. KIDNEY STONES - add kombu seaweed to the above winter tonic.

5. BED-WETTING - include black beans in the diet regularly.

CHESTNUT

Nature / Taste: warm, sweet and salty

Actions: tonifies the kidneys, strengthens digestion, fortifies the Chi, arrests cough

Conditions: weak kidney Chi, back pain, weak lower extremities, frequent urination, nausea, burping, hiccups, chronic bronchitis, cough, asthma, diarrhea

Folk Remedies:

1. DIARRHEA - grind to flour and boil for 10 - 15 minutes, then consume the porridge.

2. CHRONIC COUGH, BRONCHITIS - eat steamed chestnuts and drink chestnut leaf tea.

3. NAUSEA, HICCUPS, GASTRITIS - charcoal and powder the membrane (not the shell) and cook about 1.5 - 3 grams into rice porridge.

4. KIDNEY WEAKNESS, BACK OR LEG PAIN, FREQUENT URINATION - daily eat 2 raw chestnuts, 1 in the morning and 1 in the evening; chew thoroughly.

5. SPLINTERS, TRAUMAS, SORES - mash raw chestnuts and apply to the affected area to draw out splinter or pus, reduce pain and stop bleeding.

FILBERT (HAZEL NUT)

Nature / Taste: neutral and sweet

Actions: fortifies Chi, strengthens digestion

Conditions: diarrhea, lack of appetite

Folk Remedies

1. DIARRHEA - roast filberts and grind into meal; take 1 teaspoon twice daily with jujube date tea.

2. LACK OF APPETITE - grind raw filberts into a meal; take 1 teaspoon twice daily with tea made from citrus peels.

KIDNEY BEAN

Nature / Taste: neutral and sweet

Actions: strengthens digestion, promotes elimination, diuretic

Conditions: swelling, difficulty urinating, diarrhea

Folk Remedies:

1. SWELLING DUE TO NEPHRITIS - make a strong soup with 1/2 cup beans to 5 cups of water, cooked down to 1 cup.

2. CHRONIC DIARRHEA - roast kidney beans, then cook with rice water (the soaking water) to make a tea.

LENTIL

Nature / Taste: slightly warm and sweet

Actions: harmonize digestion, strengthen the Stomach, descend rebellious Chi, clear summer heat

Conditions: cholera, vomiting, diarrhea, dysentery

Folk Remedies
1. SUMMER DIARRHEA, DYSENTERY - grind lentils into meal and mix with rice porridge and eat.

2. HEAT STROKE WITH FEVER, RESTLESSNESS, AND DIFFICULT URINATION - eat cool lentil soup

LOTUS SEED

Nature / Taste: neutral and sweet

Action: strengthens kidneys, astringent, nutritive tonic

Conditions: kidney weakness, frequent urination, seminal emission, diarrhea

Folk Remedies:
1. NUTRITIVE TONIC - A delicious winter tonic soup can be made by boiling together lotus seeds, azuki (red) beans, and pearl barley; add a dash of honey before serving.

2. FREQUENT URINATION, SEMINAL EMISSION, DIARRHEA - cook lotus seeds and cubes of sweet potato in a rice porridge

MUNG BEAN

Nature / Taste: very cool and sweet

Actions: clears heat, detoxifies, quenches thirst, promotes urination, reduces swelling, aids edema in the lower limbs, counteracts toxins

Conditions: edema, conjunctivitis, diabetes, dysentery, summer heat problems, heatstroke, dehydration, food poisoning from spoiled food, carbuncles

Contraindications: Not for cold conditions. Females should avoid mung beans if trying to get pregnant.

Folk Remedies:
1. DYSENTERY - take 5 parts mung beans to 1 part black pepper; grind to a powder and take 1 tablespoon 3 times daily. Usually one will notice results in 6-12 hours. The black pepper acts as an anti-bacterial agent.

2. BREAST ABSCESS AND BOILS - take 2 tablespoons mung bean powder 2 times daily in warm water.

3. HIVES AND BAD SKIN LESIONS - make mung bean juice in the blender and drink raw.

4. SUMMER HEAT PROBLEMS - make soup from mung beans, barley, and rice.

PEANUT

Nature / Taste: neutral and sweet

Actions: improves appetite, strengthens spleen, regulates blood, lubricates lungs, promotes diuresis, aids in lactation

Conditions: edema, lactostasis, blood in urine, insomnia, lack of appetite

Folk Remedies:
1. EDEMA - take peanut tea for 7 consecutive days.

2. LACK OF MILK - steam peanuts, mash, and add to soupy rice.

3. CHRONIC COUGH - combine peanuts, jujube dates, and honey; make tea and take twice daily.

4. CHRONIC NEPHRITIS - combine peanuts and red dates; make tea and eat the solids. Take for 1 week.

5. INSOMNIA - boil peanut tea, take in the evening.

6. HYPERTENSION - take peanut shells and boil tea or grind into powder and take with warm water; take 3 times daily for at least 20 days.

PEA

Nature / Taste: neutral and sweet

Actions: strengthens digestion, strengthens spleen and stomach, promotes diuresis, lubricates intestines

Conditions: indigestion, edema, constipation

Folk Remedies:
1. EDEMA - roast peas until dry, powder and take with warm water.

2. INDIGESTION - make blender pea juice and take with meals.

PINE NUT

Nature / Taste: warm and sweet

Actions: lubricates lungs, stops cough, lubricates intestines, promotes body fluids

Conditions: dry cough, constipation

Contraindications: Not to be used in diarrhea, seminal emission, or any mucus conditions.

Folk Remedies:

1. DRY COUGH - grind walnuts and pine nuts, add honey and slowly cook over low flame until thick; take 2 teaspoons with warm water.

2. CONSTIPATION - eat pine nuts with rice porridge.

PUMPKIN SEED

Nature / Taste: cold and sweet

Actions: anti-parasitic, diuretic

Conditions: intestinal worms and parasites, swelling, diabetes, prostate problems

Folk Remedies:

1. INTESTINAL WORMS - roast and powder pumpkin seeds, then mix with honey and take twice daily. Or eat a large handful 2 - 3 times per day.

2. SWELLING AFTER PREGNANCY, DIABETES - make a tea from roasted pumpkin seeds.

3. PROSTATE PROBLEMS - eat a large handful of pumpkin seeds 2 times daily.

SESAME SEED (BROWN)

Nature / Taste: slightly warm and sweet

Actions: nourishes liver and kidneys, lubricates intestines, blackens gray hair, tonifies the body overall, benefits skin

Conditions: backache, weakness, premature graying, ringing in the ears, blurry vision, dizziness, constipation, dry cough, blood in the urine, tonic for older people, weak knees

Contraindications: Always grind sesame seeds because the tough cell wall makes them indigestible whole.

Folk Remedies:

1. WEAKNESS CONDITIONS, CONSTIPATION - grind sesame seeds to a meal, mix with honey to make a paste; take 2 teaspoons 2 times daily.

2. DRY COUGH AND ASTHMA - roast sesame seeds, grind to a meal and add ginger juice and honey. Take 1 teaspoon 3 times daily.

SESAME SEED (BLACK)

Nature / Taste: neutral and sweet

Actions: tonify liver and kidney, harmonize the blood, lubricate the intestines, restore hair color, nourish Yin, promotes lactation

Conditions: chronic constipation, premature balding or greying, chronic arthritis, joint inflammation, cough

Folk Remedies

1. CHRONIC CONSTIPATION - grind into a meal and mix with honey and form small chewable balls, about 6 grams each. Take one 3 times a day with rice wine.

2. PREMATURE BALDING OR GREYING - grind to a meal black sesames and black beans, and cook with rice milk. Take once daily for at least 3 months.

3. CHRONIC COUGH, ASTHMA - grind equal parts black sesame and apricot kernel; take 1 teaspoon with warm water 3 times a day.

SUNFLOWER SEED

Nature / Taste: neutral and sweet

Actions: subdues liver, lowers blood pressure, relieves dysentery, resolves pus, moisten intestines

Conditions: headache, dizziness, liver fire rising, bloody dysentery, intestinal worms

Folk Remedies:

1. HEADACHE OR DIZZINESS - grind the seeds and take with honey and warm water before bed.

2. HYPERTENSION - take sunflower seed meal with celery juice.

3. BLOODY DYSENTERY - cook the seeds with water for 1 hour, add honey; drink the liquid and eat the seeds.

SOY BEAN

Nature / Taste: cool and sweet

Actions: clears heat, detoxifies, eases urination, lubricates lungs and intestines, provides an excellent protein food

Conditions: lung and stomach heat, dry skin, ferocious appetite, stomach or mouth ulcers, swollen gums, diarrhea, constipation, general heat problems

Contraindications: Do not eat soy beans raw; they cannot be digested.

Folk Remedies:

1. HEAT CONDITIONS - drink soy milk or eat tofu. Soy milk is easily made by blending soaked soybeans with a larger volume of water; strain off the *milk* and bring to a boil for about 20 minutes; sweeten to taste. To make tofu curdle the soy milk with calcium sulfate, nigari, or lemon juice; strain and press the solids into a block.

2. DIARRHEA - charcoal soybeans and grind to a powder; take 1 teaspoon 3 times daily.

3. HABITUAL CONSTIPATION - boil tea from soybeans and drink 4 times daily.

TOFU (SOY BEAN CURD)

Nature / Taste: cool and sweet

Actions: clears heat, lubricates dryness, promotes body fluids, detoxifies, strengthens spleen and stomach

Conditions: chronic dysentery, malaria, lung tuberculosis, anemia, leukorrhea, irregular menstruation

Folk Remedies:

1. CHRONIC DYSENTERY - stir fry tofu with vinegar.

2. MALARIA - stir fry tofu with vinegar; take 3 hours prior to the onset of symptoms.

3. LUNG TUBERCULOSIS - combine tofu and the herb, Alismatis root; boil, and eat the tofu. Take daily for 2 months.

4. ANEMIA - take frozen tofu that has been thawed, mix with egg white, until the egg white has soaked into the tofu; cook and eat daily for 1 month.

5. LEUKORRHEA - steam tofu and brown sugar.

6. IRREGULAR MENSTRUATION DUE TO COLD-NESS - stew together tofu, lamb, and ginger.

To reduce the cool nature of tofu, press out the extra water, marinate with ginger and garlic, then bake. This would be more suitable for conditions of cold or dampness. Baked tofu is widely available in Oriental and health food markets.

WALNUT

Nature / Taste: slightly warm and sweet

Actions: tonifies kidneys, strengthens back, astringes lungs, relieves asthma, lubricates intestines, aids erratic or rebellious Chi, reduces cholesterol

Conditions: kidney deficiency, impotence, sexual dysfunctions, infertility, frequent urination, back and leg pain, stones in the urinary tract, cough, constipation, neurasthenia

Folk Remedies:

1. IMPOTENCY AND KIDNEY WEAKNESS - eat 20 walnuts a day for 1 month.

2. BACK PAIN AND COLD TYPE ARTHRITIS - take walnut meal with warm wine (preferably red wine).

3. KIDNEY STONES - take 120 grams (approximately 2-3 cups) walnuts, grind to a meal and add 120 grams brown sugar; roast with sesame oil. Take 1/4 of the mixture 4 times a day.

4. NEURASTHENIA - take equal portions of walnuts, sesame seeds, and dried mulberries, mash together to a paste; roll small pills and take 3 pills 3 times daily.

5. COUGH, CONSTIPATION - grind walnuts into meal and mix with honey. Take 2 tablespoons daily in warm water.

WINTER MELON SEED

Nature / Taste: cool and bland

Actions: promotes diuresis, resolves mucus, stops cough, clears heat, detoxifies

Conditions: coughing of blood, constipation, intestinal abscess (appendicitis), edema, leukorrhea

Folk Remedies:

1. COUGHING OF BLOOD, CONSTIPATION, AND IN-TESTINAL ABSCESS - make tea from the seeds.

2. EDEMA AND LEUKORRHEA - grind seeds into meal and take 1 teaspoon with warm water 3 times daily.

3. EDEMA IN THE SUMMER - cook soup with winter melon peel (purchased dry), winter melon seed, mung beans and pearl barley.

4. COUGHING BLOOD - make tea from winter melon seed, pearl barley and fresh lotus root.

MEAT, FISH, POULTRY & ANIMAL PRODUCTS

Meat, fish, poultry and eggs should always be properly cooked and never eaten raw. Seek producers that do not use drugs or inhumane treatment on the animals.

BEEF

Nature / Taste: warm and sweet

Actions: tonifies Chi and blood, strengthens spleen and stomach, dispels dampness, relieves edema, strengthens bones and tendons

Conditions: edema, abdominal distention and fullness, weak back and knees, deficient stomach and spleen

Contraindications: Not to be used with any type of skin lesions, hepatitis, or any type of kidney inflammation.

Folk Remedies:

1. DEFICIENCIES OF BLOOD, CHI, SPLEEN - take cooked ground beef and soak it in hot water for 10 minutes; drink the juice.

2. EDEMA OR CHRONIC DIARRHEA - stew beef in water for 2 hours; drink the liquid.

CHICKEN

Nature / Taste: warm and sweet

Actions: tonifies Chi, nourishes blood, aids kidney deficiency, benefits spleen and stomach

Conditions: postpartum weakness, weakness in old people, cold-type arthritis, weakness after illness or blood loss

Contraindications: Do not eat chickens that are force fed chemical pellets and injected with steroids and antibiotics. These type of chickens can cause a variety of health problems, including sterility, early female puberty, disharmony in the menstrual cycle, male impotence, to name a few. Also, chicken is not to be consumed by those with *heat type* cancers such as leukemia, or when there are heat symptoms such as red tongue, fever, and extreme thirst.

Folk Remedies:
1. WEAKNESS OR ANEMIA - cook 1 chicken with 1 ounce Dang Gui (Angelica sinensis), and 6 1/2 c. water. Simmer together for 1 hour. The darker meat birds such as the Chinese black chicken are the most tonifying.

TURKEY is also warm but not so tonifying as CHICKEN.

CHICKEN EGG

Nature / Taste: cool and sweet

Actions: nourishes Yin, tonifies blood, stabilizes hyperactive fetus, lubricates dryness

Conditions: dry cough, hoarse voice, dysentery, blood and Yin deficiency, hyperactive fetus

Contraindications: Eating too many eggs is not healthy. In general, do not eat eggs fried or raw.

Folk Remedies:
1. YIN AND BLOOD DEFICIENCY - steam the eggs.

2. POSTPARTUM - eat eggs with green onions.

3. PAIN OF DYSENTERY - cook eggs with rice vinegar.

4. HYPERACTIVE FETUS - eat a hard boiled egg daily.

FISH

Nature / Taste: warm* and sweet

Actions: strengthens spleen, tonifies Chi, removes dampness, regulates blood, aids diarrhea from spleen weakness

Conditions: low energy states, hemorrhoids, postpartum excessive bleeding, itching or exuding damp type skin lesions.

Contraindications: Do not eat fish raw, as it is often loaded with parasites. Always cook fish with garlic, ginger or onion to neutralize the potential toxins.

Folk Remedies:
1. KIDNEY DEFICIENCY AND BACK PAIN - cook chicken with fish.

OCEAN FISH would be cooler than FRESHWATER FISH. Many of the ocean fishes are considered neutral. CLAMS and CRABS are cool, OYSTERS are neutral, and SHRIMP is warm. The SHELLFISH can cause rashes and other allergic reactions.

LAMB

Nature / Taste: hot and sweet

Actions: tonifies weakness, dispels cold, strengthens and nourishes Chi and blood, promotes appetite, aids lactation

Conditions: kidney deficiency causing back pain, impotence, cold conditions, deficiency conditions, postpartum blood loss, lack of milk, leukorrhea

Contraindications: Lamb is generally not consumed in summer because of its hot nature. Not to be consumed in edema, malaria, common cold, toothache or any type of heat conditions.

Folk Remedies:
1. ANEMIA, WEAKNESS, BLOOD DEFICIENCY- cook lamb with ginger and Dang Gui (Angelica sinensis). In general, the meats are traditionally prepared with such herbs as Dang Gui, jujube date, astragalus, ginger, scallions, or ginseng for problems of weakness and coldness.

MILK AND MILK PRODUCTS

Nature / Taste: neutral and sweet

Actions: strengthens weakness, nourishes Chi and blood, lubricates dryness

Conditions: nutritional deficiency, weakness, malnutrition, anemia, constipation, dryness

Contraindications: Not to be used with damp or cold conditions, or in cases of diarrhea. In general not to be used by adults or those who are strong as dairy products can then cause mucus and other disorders. As an occasional food used moderately, it should not cause a problem; however, not to be used daily. Allergy is common with this food since many adults lose the ability to digest milk sugar after infancy. Allergic reactions usually include diarrhea and bloating.

Folk Remedies:
1. WEAKNESS, MALNUTRITION - give a glass of warm milk.

PORK

Nature / Taste: slightly cold and sweet

Actions: moistens and nourishes organs, tonifies Chi, strengthens the digestion

Conditions: internal dryness, constipation, dry cough, emaciation

Contraindications: Not to be taken by fat people, those with deficient spleen and stomach, hypertension, stroke victims or those with diarrhea.

Folk Remedies:

1. CONSTIPATION, DRY COUGH - make soup with pork, carrots and lily bulbs.

2. WEAKNESS, EMACIATION - cook pork in a rice porridge.

MISCELLANEOUS FOODS, HERBS, AND BEVERAGES

ANISE SEED

Nature / Taste: warm and pungent

Actions: strengthens stomach, regulates Chi flow, harmonizes stomach, stops vomiting

Conditions: hernia, beriberi, abdominal pain, distention and gas, back pain and coldness, cold stomach

Contraindications: Not to be used in any type of heat conditions..

Folk Remedies:

1. STOMACH PAIN DUE TO COLDNESS - make anise tea and add some wine.

2. HERNIA - charcoal anise and grind to powder; add brown sugar and take with rice wine.

BARLEY MALT SYRUP

Nature / Flavor: neutral and sweet

Actions: promotes digestion, relieves food stagnation, strengthens stomach, stops lactation

Conditions: food retention (due to wheat products), epigastric fullness and distention, belching, constipation, undesirable lactation

Folk Remedies

1. FOOD RETENTION AND STOPPING LACTATION - drink barley malt in warm water until condition resolves. *RICE MALT SYRUP is neutral and sweet and has similar*

properties to barley malt, except that rice malt is better for food stagnation due to rice products

BASIL

Nature / Taste: warm and pungent

Actions: induces sweating, harmonizes stomach, antidote for seafood poisoning

Conditions: wind-cold, vomiting, diarrhea, seafood poisoning

Folk Remedies:
1. COMMON COLD - boil tea from basil, ginger, and green onions.
2. DIARRHEA, VOMITING, SEAFOOD POISONING - boil basil tea.

BLACK FUNGUS (WOOD EARS)

Nature / Taste: neutral, slightly toxic raw, and sweet

Actions: nourishes stomach, calms spirit, lubricates dryness, promotes blood flow, removes stagnation

Conditions: blood stagnation such as tumor, especially uterine, abnormal uterine bleeding, bloody stools, hemorrhoids, constipation, hypertension

Contraindications: Not to be used by pregnant women.

Folk Remedies:
1. HYPERTENSION, BLOODY STOOLS, AND HEMORRHOIDS - take black fungus and dried persimmon, add some honey, cook, and eat once a day.
2. ABNORMAL BLEEDING, ANEMIA - boil tea from black fungus and Chinese dates.

3. DYSENTERY - take 10 grams fresh black fungus with warm water 2 times daily.

4. TUMORS OF THE VISCERAS AND FEMALE ORGANS - make tea from black fungus and peach kernel, and drink.

BLACK PEPPER

Nature / Flavor: hot and pungent

Actions: warms digestion, dispels internal cold, antidote to food poisoning

Conditions: stomachache due to cold, diarrhea, food poisoning

Folk Remedies:
1. FOOD POISONING - mix 1 t. black pepper with rice porridge and grated ginger and drink as much as possible.

BROWN SUGAR (TURBINADO SUGAR)

Nature / Taste: warm and sweet

Actions: strengthens digestion, lubricates the lungs, stops cough, warms up the body

Conditions: dry cough, poor digestion, coldness

Folk Remedies:
1. STOMACH PAINS, ULCER PAINS - mix a spoonful into warm water and drink to arrest pain.

2. DRY COUGH, SORE THROAT - grate carrots and mix with brown sugar. Refrigerate over night, then consume the next day.

Contraindications: Not to be consumed in excess. Can lead to mucus and dampness in the body.

WHITE SUGAR is sweet and cold; it lubricates the lungs, treats dry cough, and promotes the healing of bed sores, ulcerations and burns when used externally. Apply sugar to the lesion and rebandage every 3 - 5 days. The same contraindications for brown sugar apply to white sugar.

CARDAMON SEED

Nature / Taste: warm and pungent

Actions: warms the digestion, resolves dampness, invigorates the flow of Chi, stops vomiting

Conditions: dampness, diarrhea, nausea, vomiting, stomach ulcers, abdominal distention and fullness

Folk Remedies:
1. STOMACH AND DUODENAL ULCERS - on an empty stomach every morning, drink cardamon and fresh ginger root tea.

2. ABDOMINAL PAIN AND DISTENTION - make tea from cardamon, cloves and orange peel. Drink 3 times daily.

3. NAUSEA AND DIARRHEA - stir 1 teaspoon cardamon powder into 1 cup of warm water and drink 3 times a day.

CAROB POD

Nature / Taste: warm and sweet

Actions: soothes and calms the spirit

Conditions: used as an alternative to chocolate, and for caffeine addiction

Contraindications: Eating carob to excess will cause agitation.

Folk Remedies:
1. CHOCOLATE SUBSTITUTE - use powdered carob pods.

CINNAMON

Nature / Taste: hot, pungent and sweet

Actions: strengthens stomach, warms any coldness in the body, stops pain

Conditions: common cold, abdominal pain due to cold stagnation, lack of appetite due to cold stomach, low back pain

Contraindications: Not to be used in pregnancy.

Folk Remedies:
1. POSTPARTUM ABDOMINAL PAIN - boil tea with cinnamon and brown sugar.

2. PREMENSTRUAL SYNDROME, INCLUDING LOWER ABDOMINAL PAIN AND BLOATING PRIOR TO MENSTRUATION - make tea from cinnamon and hawthorn berries.

3. GAS PAIN IN STOMACH AREA - take 1/2 teaspoon cinnamon powder with lukewarm water, 2 times daily.

CLOVE

Nature / Taste: warm and pungent

Actions: warm the middle, dispel internal cold, reverse rebellious Chi, warms the kidneys, stops pain

Conditions: stomachache due to cold, vomiting, nausea, belching, hiccupping, toothache

Folk Remedies
1. VOMITING, NAUSEA, BELCHING - drink 1 teaspoon clove powder in warm water.
2. TOOTHACHE - place clove above or below the affected tooth on the gum until pain is relieved.

COFFEE

Nature / Taste: warm, sweet and bitter

Actions: stimulating, diuretic, promotes elimination

Conditions: mild swelling, constipation, hypersomnia, lethargy, mental cloudiness, conditions that require stimulation

Contraindications: This beverage is a very addictive substance. Avoid in high blood pressure, insomnia, nervousness, and stomach ulcers or acidity; coffee is easier on the stomach if taken with milk or soy milk. Always exercise moderation in its use. Avoid during pregnancy.

FENNEL SEED

Nature / Taste: warm and pungent

Actions: unblocks and regulates Chi, strengthens stomach, dispels cold, stops pain, stimulates peristalsis

Conditions: stomachache, hernia, abdominal discomfort, coldness in the stomach, colic in babies

Folk Remedies:
1. HERNIA - boil tea from fennel seeds, black pepper, cinnamon, and orange peel. Externally apply warming liniment and heating pad.

GINGER ROOT (FRESH)

Nature / Taste: warm and pungent

Actions: promotes sweating, anti-toxin, antidote for seafood poisoning, benefits the lungs and stomach, expels pathogen

Conditions: common cold, cough due to coldness (clear or white mucus), nausea, vomiting, diarrhea, *cold type* arthritis

Folk Remedies:

1. COLDS, COUGH, VOMITING - make ginger tea.

2. DIARRHEA - apply ginger plaster to the belly.

3. BALDNESS - rub fresh ginger on the scalp.

4. ARTHRITIS - rub fresh ginger on painful areas and drink tea (not for *heat type* arthritis).

5. NAUSEA - squeeze ginger juice into some water and sip slowly until nausea is reduced.

DRIED GINGER is hot and pungent and would be used to dispel coldness. For stomach or abdominal pain, drink tea made from dried ginger and cloves.

HONEY

Nature / Taste: neutral (unless heated, then it is warm) and sweet

Actions: nourishes Yin, lubricates dryness, tonifies weakness, harmonizes, antidote to drugs, strengthens spleen

Conditions: diabetes (small amounts), constipation, ulcers, dry cough, hoarse voice, burns, cold sores

Contraindications: Not to be used in diarrhea or conditions of dampness or phlegm.

Folk Remedies:

1. ULCERS - mix ginger juice and honey and take on an empty stomach every morning.

2. BURNS - apply locally.

3. COUGH, CONSTIPATION, AND HOARSENESS - mix honey with water and/or almonds.

Try to avoid heating honey unless a warming nature is desired; heating lowers the nourishing and beneficial effects. The darker honeys are more tonifying and tend to sink to the lower parts of the body. The lighter honeys are better for upper body problems.

MOLASSES

Nature / Taste: warm and sweet

Actions: tonifies Chi, strengthens spleen, lubricates lungs, stops cough

Conditions: stomach and abdominal pain, Chi deficiency, cough

Folk Remedies:

1. STOMACH OR DUODENAL ULCERS - take 2 teaspoons molasses in lukewarm water to stop pain.

2. COUGH - dice carrots, mix with molasses and leave it overnight; take 2 teaspoons 3 times daily.

3. BED-WETTING - boil cinnamon and licorice tea, add 2 teaspoons molasses.

OLIVE

Nature / Taste: neutral, sweet, sour and astringent

Actions: clears heat, detoxifies, promotes body fluids, quenches thirst, clears lungs, benefits the throat

Conditions: whooping cough, dysentery, sore throat, dehydration, laryngitis, thirst

Folk Remedies:
1. COUGH AND DRY CONDITIONS - take olives regularly.

2. SORE, DRY THROAT AND LARYNGITIS - take 50 black, pitted olives and 3-4 cups of honey; heat over a low flame. Take 2-3 tablespoons 3 times daily, swallowing slowly.

RICE VINEGAR

Nature / Taste: warm and sour

Actions: detoxifies, invigorates blood circulation, inhibits bacteria, astringent, closes pores

Conditions: preventative for common colds, prevents invasion from external pathogens, malaria, acute arthritis, vomiting, nausea, intestinal worms, hypertension, burns, fungus infestation, bones caught in the throat, gum disease, hives, hepatitis, lung tuberculosis, lung abscess, bronchitis

Contraindications: Not to be used at the onset of a cold as it will trap the pathogens inside of the body.

Folk Remedies:
1. MALARIA - mix 30-50 c.c. of rice vinegar with 2 teaspoons baking soda; take 2 hours before the episodic attack of chills and fever.

2. ACUTE ARTHRITIS - boil 2 cups rice vinegar down to 1 cup; add green onions and boil another 5 minutes. Soak

gauze pad and apply to sore area twice daily until condition improves.

3. NAUSEA AND VOMITING - mix equal parts of rice vinegar and water and drink.

4. INTESTINAL WORMS - take rice vinegar with water on an empty stomach.

5. HYPERTENSION - soak peanuts in vinegar; eat 20 peanuts every morning.

6. BURNS - apply undiluted.

7. FISH BONES IN THE THROAT - slowly drink 1 cup vinegar, then eat something hard like bread crust.

8. GUM DISEASE - rinse mouth often with undiluted vinegar.

9. HIVES - make ginger tea, add rice vinegar and brown sugar; take twice daily.

10. HEPATITIS - soak apple-pear in vinegar; eat daily.

11. LUNG T.B. - soak garlic in rice vinegar for 2-7 days; take 1 clove 2 times daily.

12. LUNG ABSCESS - boil garlic in vinegar; take 1-2 cloves daily.

13. BRONCHITIS - combine 10 mashed garlic cloves, 1 cup vinegar, and 2 teaspoons brown sugar; take 2 teaspoons 3 times daily.

SALT

Nature / Flavor: cold, salty and slightly sweet

Actions: harmonize and promote digestion, strengthens the kidney in (small amounts), fortifies bones, tendons and teeth, brightens eyes, detoxifies, used as a natural preservative

Conditions: food poisoning, kidney weakness from lack of sodium in the diet, sore throat

Folk Remedies:
1. FOOD POISONING - for immediate relief roast salt and take with warm water which will cause vomiting to relieve condition.

2. ITCHY, INFLAMED SKIN - wash area with salt water or apply salt.

3. SORE THROAT - gargle with warm salt water several times per day.

TEA

Nature / Taste: cool, bitter and sweet

Actions: clears the head, refreshes the mind, relieves thirst and restlessness, resolves phlegm, diuretic, promote digestion, detoxifies, reduces cholesterol

Conditions: headaches, blurry vision, thirst, restlessness, foggy head, hypersomnia, food retention, dysentery, difficulty urinating, overweight

Contraindications: Avoid or minimal use with insomnia. Better not to have on an empty stomach due to tannin.

Folk Remedies
1. FOR THE ABOVE CONDITIONS, prepare tea leaves (preferably green tea) and drink as needed.

WHITE FUNGUS (SILVER EARS)

Nature / Taste: neutral and sweet

Actions: clears lung heat, strengthens spleen and stomach, promotes body fluids, tonifies Chi, invigorates blood, lubricates intestines, relieves alcohol intoxication, nourishes Yin, especially of the lungs

Conditions: cough, dry lungs, bloody sputum, irregular menstruation, arteriosclerosis, hypertension, alcohol intoxication, blood stagnation, constipation

Folk Remedies:

1. LUNG PROBLEMS, CONSTIPATION, BLOODY SPUTUM - soak white fungus 12 hours, add honey, and steam. Drink the liquid on an empty stomach. This is known as *silver ears soup*.

2. ARTERIOSCLEROSIS, HYPERTENSION, EYE HEMORRHAGE -drink *silver ears soup* before bedtime.

3. WEAKNESS AFTER LONG ILLNESS OR LOSS OF BLOOD - slowly stew white fungus, 10 Chinese dates, and either pork or chicken.

WINE

Nature / Taste: warm, pungent and sweet

Actions: promotes circulation, enhances the effect of circulatory herbs, stops pain temporarily

Conditions: arthritis, traumas, bruises, painful conditions

Contraindications: This can be a very addictive substance. In case of allergy to alcohol, avoid completely. Not good for heat conditions, and avoid during pregnancy. Do not mix wine with fatty foods.

Folk Remedies:

1. ARTHRITIS (COLD TYPE) WITH NUMBNESS AND STIFFNESS, NEURALGIA - dry stir fry black beans until the bean splits and they slightly burn; soak in good quality rice wine over night. Filter and drink a small amount twice a day.

2. TRAUMA AND PAIN - drink warm sake (rice wine), or other good quality wine for temporary relief.

3. MENSTRUAL PAIN - drink wine that was prepared with the herb Motherwort (Leonorus cardiaca) prior to the onset of period; the period will probably be a little heavier flow.

SECTION

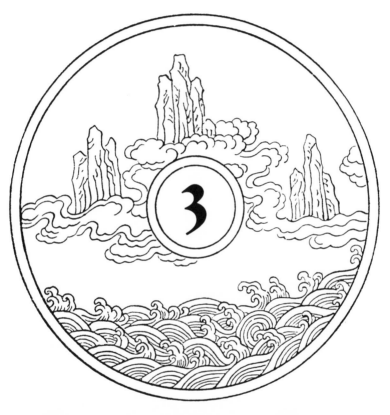

3

Remedies For Common Conditions

ACNE

This condition is characterized by skin blemishes or pimples. It can occur at any point throughout the lifetime and is often related to a hormonal imbalance. In Chinese terminology the skin is controlled by the lungs, and acne is commonly a condition of heat in the lungs. Thus, the Chinese approach to this condition is to cool the heat, cleanse the lungs, and also externally work on the healing process.

Recommendations: squash, cucumbers, watermelon, winter melon, celery, carrots, cabbage, beet tops, dandelions, aloe vera, mulberry leaf, carrot tops, lettuce, potato, cherries, papaya, pear, persimmon, raspberries, buckwheat, alfalfa sprouts, millet, brown rice, mung beans, plenty of water

Remedies:

1. Blend a cucumber, apply externally; leave on for 20 minutes then wash off.

2. Apply plain, low fat, no chemicals yogurt; leave on for 20 minutes then wash off.

3. Rub watermelon rind on the acne.

4. Apply aloe vera.

5. Eat watermelon or drink watermelon juice.

6. Drink dandelion and beet top tea.

7. Drink lukewarm water with 2 teaspoons of honey every morning on an empty stomach. This effectively lubricates the intestines. If one does not evacuate the intestines regularly, the toxins either end up in the liver or coming out on the skin.

8. Boil raspberries to a concentrate and wash area with it.

9. Roast buckwheat, grind to powder and mix with rice vinegar into a paste, then apply to area.

10. For oozing acne condition, cover area with pearl barley powder over night, wash off with water; or, mix pearl barley powder with aloe vera gel into a paste and leave on area over night, then wash off with water.

11. Drink tea made from carrot tops, carrots, and beet tops.

12. For infected acne, apply dandelion poultice to the area.

Avoid: fried foods, fatty or oily foods, spicy foods, coffee, alcohol, sugar, smoking, stress, constipation, make-up, washing with chemicals or soap (wash with cool water)*, chocolate, ice cream, soft drinks, dairy foods, emotional stress, red meat, shellfish, bamboo shoots, white mushrooms *If the face is dirty, steam it with hot water to induce sweating, then wash with cold water.*

ACQUIRED IMMUNE DEFICIENCY SYNDROME (A.I.D.S.)

A.I.D.S. is a chronic retro-viral infection with the human immunodeficiency virus (H.I.V.) in a susceptible host, which produces severe defects in the cells. There is a reduction of part of the immune system called the helper T cells. This leaves the patient vulnerable to many opportunistic infections and unusual cancers. The H.I.V. virus is transmitted via sexual contact, exposure to infected blood or perinatal exposure. Prominent symptoms include diarrhea, sweating, weight loss, neuropathy and wasting away. Aggressive infections, like pneumonia and candidiasis, prove to be life threatening, when the immune system is so compromised.

Recommendations: pearl barley, Shitake mushroom, Ling Zhi (Ganoderma) mushroom, garlic, white and black fungus, brussel sprouts, bitter melon, squash, pumpkin,

pumpkin seed, yam, apricot kernel, Chinese cucumber (Trichosanthis), water chestnut, mung bean, black bean, ginkgo nut, loquat, dandelion greens, egg yolk, jujube date, wild yam, green tea, daikon radish, lotus root, lotus seed, hawthorn berry

Remedies

1. Make brown rice porridge with pearl barley, mung beans, yams and lotus seeds.

2. Soak dried Shitake mushrooms and /or white fungus, black fungus, and Ling Zhi mushrooms overnight. Boil for 10 minutes in the soaking water. Then liquify in blender along with organic carrot tops. Drink on empty stomach daily.

3. Make tea by simmering for 30 minutes, Chinese cucumber and jujube dates. Drink 3 cups per day. 4. Make juice with fresh water chestnut, lotus root, dandelion greens and fresh ginger.

5. Grind together apricot kernels, pumpkin seeds, nori seaweed, sesame seeds, cardamon and a pinch of salt. Use generously as seasoning over vegetables and grains.

6. Liquify fresh ginger root and aloe vera leaf (use only the soft center, peeling away the hard outer part). Drink 1 cup daily.

7. Consult a Chinese Herbalist/Acupuncturist for a Chinese herb formula.

Avoid: dairy, alcohol, coffee, sugar, fatty or fried foods, overly spicy foods, cold and raw foods, tomato, eggplant, bell peppers, shellfish

ALLERGY AND INTOLERANCE

Allergy is an acquired hypersensitivity to a substance that does not normally cause a body reaction. The allergenic substance may be pollen, smog, dust, certain chemicals in the air, chlorine, or certain food substances which elicit a sometimes violent body response. This condition is characterized by nasal congestion, tearing, sneezing, wheezing, coughing, itching, skin rash and eruptions, dizziness and nausea.

Recommendations: ginger, onions, garlic, bamboo shoots, cabbage, beets, beet top tea, carrots, leafy greens, yams, organic chicken gizzards

Remedies:

1. Drink ginger tea to induce sweating.

2. Drink beet top tea as a water source.

Avoid: wheat, citrus fruits, chocolate, shellfish, dairy products, eggs, potatoes, polluted meats, polluted air, and constipation

ANOREXIA AND BULIMIA

Anorexia is medically defined as a lack of appetite for food or a hysterical avoidance of food. This condition is particularly prevalent among young American women obsessed with being thin. There is usually an extreme loss of weight, no menstruation, fatigue, depression, and hypoglycemic patterns. Closely related to anorexia is bulimia, a condition in which one binges then purges, usually by vomiting. Emotional factors play a large part in both of these conditions.

Recommendations: bell pepper, cilantro, mustard greens, green onions, garlic, cinnamon, ginger, pumpkin, yam, beans, corn, barley, rice, persimmons, potatoes

Remedies:

1. For anorexia, prepare tea from green onions, garlic, cinnamon or ginger, to warm the stomach and stimulate digestive juices.

2. For anorexia, prepare soup from pumpkin, yam, beans, potatoes, corn, barley or vegetables.

3. For anorexia, prepare soupy rice.

4. For bulimia, give foods that bring rebellious Chi down such as persimmons, cloves, potatoes, prune or plum tea, and mineral herbs such as oyster shell or mother of pearl shell tea.

5. For anorexia, dry fry bell pepper and black pepper.

ARTHRITIS

Arthritis is an inflammation of the joints characterized by pain, redness, swelling, stiffness and hot sensation in the joints. Chinese medicine differentiates the following 4 types of arthritis. Often we observe 2 or 3 types of arthritis occurring simultaneously, such as cold and damp types together. In such cases, choose foods that aid each condition and are not contraindicated for either type. Herbal therapy can be of great benefit in cleaning out the joints, improving the circulation, and reducing the pain. Acupuncture is one of the most effective treatments for arthritis, although progress is sometimes slow.

1. COLD TYPE ARTHRITIS
This type is characterized by sharp, stabbing pain in a fixed

location and coldness in the joints. The pain is relieved by heat such as a warming liniment, sunshine, or a heating pad. Usually this type individual would have a pale complexion.

Recommendations: garlic, green onions, pepper, black beans, sesame seeds, chicken, lamb, mustard greens, ginger, a small amount of rice wine (if individual does not have hypertension), 10-20 minutes of fresh air and sunshine daily, spicy foods, grapes, grape vine, parsnip

Remedies:
1. Rub garlic or ginger on the painful areas. Or moxa could be burned on ginger over the painful areas.

2. Drink scallion tea and rub on the painful areas.

3. Rub rice wine on the painful areas as well as consuming 1 shot glassful in the evening.

4. Drink grape vine tea added to red wine.

5. Make tea from parsnip, cinnamon, black pepper, and dried ginger.

Avoid: cold foods, raw foods, cold weather elements

2. WIND TYPE ARTHRITIS
This type of arthritis is characterized by pain that shifts locations, comes and goes suddenly (much like the wind does), and sometimes causes dizziness.

Recommendations: snake meat (from non-poisonous ones), scallions, grapes (not wine), grape vine and mulberry vine tea, black beans, most grains, and plenty of leafy vegetables

Avoid: meats, shellfish, sugar, alcohol, smoking, and all stimulants

3. DAMP TYPE ARTHRITIS

This is characterized by heavy feeling extremities, stiffness, swelling, dull aching pain that lingers and sluggishness. Most obese people tend to be *damp.*

Recommendations: barley, mung beans, mustard greens, red beans, millet, sweet rice wine with meals, cornsilk tea, diuretic foods and herbs

Remedies:
1. Cook together barley, mung beans and red beans.
2. Drink cornsilk tea freely.

Avoid: cold foods, raw foods, dairy products

4. HEAT TYPE ARTHRITIS

This is characterized by red, swollen, painful, hot joints, general disability, and usually acute onset.

Recommendations: plenty of fresh fruits and vegetables, dandelion, cabbage, mung beans, winter melon, soybean sprouts

Remedies:
1. Apply poultices of crushed dandelion greens, changing every 2 hours.

Avoid: spicy foods, alcohol, smoking, all types of stress, green onions

ASTHMA

Asthma is characterized by wheezing or difficulty breathing due to the bronchials (branches) of the lungs becoming clogged with waste products, or constriction due to spasms, or swelling of the bronchials. Asthma may be triggered by an allergy to food, air pollution, cold air, heart weakness, previous lung damage, mental or physical fatigue, emotional disturbance, or hormonal imbalance. In the case of a weak heart, the heart is not strong enough to push the blood through the lungs to be oxygenated, and the blood back flows into the lungs. In this case there will be edema and bruising also.

Chinese medicine divides asthma into 2 types: *hot type,* characterized by rapid, coarse breathing, yellow, sticky mucus, fever, and red face; and *cold type,* characterized by white, clear, or foamy mucus, cold extremities, and pale face. The remedies listed would be useful to either type. During times of remission from asthma attack, one would seek to nourish the lungs and kidneys.

Recommendations: apricot kernels, almonds, walnuts, basil, carrots, pumpkins, winter melon, sunflower seeds, loofa squash, figs, daikon, litchi (lychee) fruit, tangerines, loquats, honey, molasses, mustard greens, sesame seeds, placenta* and umbilical cord*

These substances are not so easily obtainable in America, and only those from a healthy mother source are desirable.

Remedies:

1. Egg yolk oil. This is made as follows: take 20 hard boiled egg yolks; slowly heat in a dry pan, mashing them until the oil comes out. When the yolk has blackened, separate the egg yolk oil. Since it is very strong tasting, it is best taken in gelatin capsules, 2 after meals, 3 times daily. Continue this remedy for 15-30 days.

2. Mix 1/2 cup fig juice with 1/2 cup lukewarm water and drink daily.

3. Cut the top out of a small winter melon, remove the seeds, fill with molasses, close the top up with cheesecloth and steam. Consume daily for 7 days.

4. Take an unpeeled orange, stick a chopstick through it, roast until the peel blackens. Remove the peel and eat the insides; one orange daily for 7 days.

5. Bake squid bone until crisp; grind to a powder and take 1 teaspoon with honey daily for 7 days.

6. Drink apricot kernel tea.

7. Drink fresh fig juice 3 times daily.

Avoid: mucus producing foods, cold foods, fruits, salads, all shellfish, dairy products, watermelon, bananas, mung beans, salty foods, cold weather, and especially ice cream

CANCER

According to Chinese Medicine, cancer is an abnormalgrowth of tissue that results from some sort of stagnation, of Chi, blood, mucus, or body fluids. The stagnation can be caused by some external irritant such as cigarette smoke or chemicalized foods or by strong emotions. When the body is irritated over a long period of time, it reacts to the irritant by growing to protect itself. However, at a certain point the cell growth becomes abnormal and uncontrollable and cancer cells result. Strong emotions lead to Chi stagnation which in turn can lead to stagnation of blood, mucus or body fluids.

The Western approach to cancer is to kill the cancercells with harsh chemicals, radiation, or surgery. However, these methods also harm the healthy cells. The Chinese approach to cancer is to support the body so that it can combat the cancer cells itself. The cancer is considered to be a toxin in the body, thus a detoxifying diet is also utilized.

126

Recommendations: seaweed, Shitake mushrooms, figs, beets, beet tops, papayas, mung beans, licorice, sea cucumbers, carrots, garlic, walnuts, litchi fruits, mulberries, asparagus, pumpkins, burdock, dandelion greens, white fungus, taro roots, pearl barley, grains, plenty of fresh fruits and vegetables

Remedies:

1. Blend Shitake or Ling Zhi mushrooms and white fungus, boil and drink the soup 3 times daily.

2. Boil together mung beans, pearl barley, azuki beans, and figs. This makes a delicious dessert that will aid appetite and sustain the energy level.

3. Make tea from dandelion, burdock, and chrysanthemum flowers; you may also add beet tops or carrot tops. Drink this as the regular beverage every day.

4. Always wash commercially grown fruits and vegetables in salt water to neutralize the chemicals.

5. Take garlic and seaweed, slightly stir fried in water.

6. Drink carrot and celery juice.

7. Make blender juice from a mixture of fresh vegetables and take warm.

8. For breast cancer, make tea from asparagus and dandelion and apply poultice to breast.

9. For breast tumor, charcoal the pumpkin *cap* into powder; take 1 t. of powder in 1 shot of rice wine 2 times daily.

10. Make tea from seaweed (any variety), peach kernel and green orange peels. Externally for visible tumors, make poultice from seaweed, ginger and dandelion, and apply locally.

Avoid: meat (if patient cannot handle vegetarian diet a little fish could be eaten), chicken, coffee, cinnamon, anise, pepper, dairy products, spicy foods (except garlic), high fat foods, cooked oils, chemical additives, moldy foods, smoking, constipation, stress, and all irritations

CANDIDA YEAST INFECTION

This condition is becoming fairly common in modern society, primarily due to the widespread, long term use of antibiotics which severely weaken the immune system. Everyone has the candida yeast living in their bodies; however, only when disharmony and weakness occur do we have systemic yeast infections develop. The symptoms can include chronic fatigue, chronic infections, primarily in the skin, bowels, bladder, vagina, and throat; diarrhea or constipation, headaches, bloating, and poor digestion. When the immune system is weakened through overwork, too much sex, or stress, the candida flares up and the body can no longer control it. In the case of A.I.D.S., candida infection can become life threatening.

Recommendations: dandelions, beet tops, carrot tops, barley, garlic, rice vinegar, mung beans, citrus fruits

Avoid: sugar, excessive fruits, yeast containing foods, processed foods, cheese, fermented foods, soy sauce, smoking, alcohol, caffeine, and constipation.

CATARACT

This is a condition that usually affects older people in which the lens of the eye becomes cloudy and there is decreased visual acuity. It may be accompanied by dizziness, vertigo, fatigue, and lower back pain. Western medicine treats cataract by surgically removing the lens.

Recommendations: chrysanthemum, cilantro, spinach, cloves, water chestnuts, yams, lycii berries, black beans. Exercise the eyes regularly and get plenty of oxygen into the bloodstream.

Remedies:

1. Stuff nose with fresh cilantro and inhale the aroma; do this 3 times daily.

2. Cook spinach with no spices and eat daily.

3. Steam the eyes over boiling spinach.

4. Grind cloves into a very fine powder and add a little milk to make an ointment. Apply to eyes 3 to 5 times daily.

5. Make fresh water chestnut juice and use as an eye drop.

6. Make tea from clam shells, orange peels, lycii berries, and chrysanthemum. Drink 3 times daily for at least 2 weeks.

7. Mash together black beans, sesames, yams,and walnuts then add a little honey and eat 1 T. 2 times daily for 1 month

Avoid: any type of spices (very important), salt, garlic, eyestrain, constipation

CHRONIC BLADDER INFECTION

This is a common condition in women, characterized by painful or burning urination, the feeling that there is still urine left in the bladder after urinating; fever, low back ache. If this condition occurs in a man it is a warning sign of something more serious such as venereal disease or cancer. Women are prone to chronic bladder infections because of the short length of their urethras. In Chinese terminology it is a condition of damp heat.

Recommendations: watermelon, pears, carrots, celery, corn, mung beans, cornsilk, squash, wheat, water chestnuts, barley, red beans, millet, oranges, cantaloupe, grapes, strawberries, lotus roots, loquats, plenty of water, and in general cooling and diuretic foods

Remedies:
1. Drink watermelon and pear juice 3 times daily.
2. Drink carrot and celery juice 3 times daily.
3. Drink cornsilk tea freely.
4. Eat squash soup for at least 7 days.
5. Eat steamed lotus root and water chestnuts 2 times daily.
6. Drink blended mung bean juice.
7. Drink fresh strawberry juice.
8. Drink tea made from wheat and pearl barley.

Avoid: heavy proteins, meat, dairy products, onions, scallions, ginger, black pepper, alcohol

CHRONIC BRONCHITIS

This is a common condition in older people, commonly due to a lowered immunity. It often occurs during winter and spring. Main symptoms include cough, mucus, shortness of breath, and fullness in the chest.

Recommendations: carrots, apricot kernels, persimmons, white fungus, pears, honey, jellyfish, ginger, water chestnuts, yams, sweet potatoes, Chinese red or black dates, daikon radish, walnuts, papaya, peach kernels, lotus roots, seaweed, betel nut, white pepper, loquat leaves, lily bulbs, pine nuts, mulberry leaves, chrysanthemum, ginkgo nuts, basil seeds, pumpkins, taro, winter melon seeds. Always try to keep warm.

Remedies:

1. Take carrots and apricot kernels cooked with rice porridge. Take 3 times daily for 30 days.

2. Take white fungus and rock sugar, steam and eat 2 - 3 times daily for 1 month.

3. Take 2 - 3 pears, remove core and fill with honey and eat before bed every day for 1 month.

4. Take jellyfish and water chestnut to make soup.

5. Take ginger, apricot kernel, pine nuts, and walnuts; mash, add rock sugar, and steam. Eat 2 - 3 T. twice daily for at least 14 days.

6. Make juice from pineapple and lemon; drink before meals for immediate relief.

7. Take 3 dried persimmons boiled in 2 c. water, reduced to 1 c., add some honey, drink 2 - 3 times daily.

8. Take daikon, add maltose and steam. Eat 2 - 3 times daily for relief within 1 week.

9. Take papaya, peeled, add honey and steam.

10. Grind seaweed into powder, add honey and make into pills and take 1 t. 2 - 3 times daily after meals.

11. Boil tea from betel nuts, drink as your water for 1 month.

12. Take carrots, white pepper, ginger, and dried orange peels and make tea. Drink 2 c. daily.

13. Take 1 T. honey and 1 T. sesame oil, warm in pan and take for immediate relief.

14. Cut banana into small pieces and cook with rock sugar until sugar melts. Take 1 - 2 pieces of banana every evening for 1 week.

15. Use seed from such vegetables as daikon, basil, spinach, and make tea, adding honey.

16. Take 1 T. molasses and 1/2 T. raw ginger juice with warm water 2 - 3 times daily.

17. Use fresh, yellow chrysanthemum flowers and boil into a thick juice; take regularly.

18. Mash cooked taro root and add honey.

19. Take raw eggplant juice (especially good for blood in the mucus).

Avoid: overworking, getting chilled, stimulating foods, spicy foods, smoking, alcohol, caffeine, cold drinks

CHRONIC FATIGUE SYNDROME

This syndrome consists of a set of variable symptoms including chronic or recurrent fatigue, sore throat, tender lymph nodes, headaches, muscle pains, and general depression. Often the patient has flu-like symptoms that extend for a long period of time. Most Chronic fatigue patients are observed to have undergone prolonged stress, repeated infections, and often become overwhelmed by life's simple demands. Conditions like herpes, candida and hypoglycemia compound the situation. Patient is advised to seek lifestyle corrections, like reducing stress, resting more, and gentle exercise.

Recommendations: winter melon, pumpkin, pumpkin seed, yam, sweet potato, lima bean, black bean, soy bean, strawberry, watermelon, azuki bean, pineapple, chestnut, papaya, figs garlic, onion, scallion, ginger daikon radish, pearl barley, lotus seed, white fungus, egg white, cabbage, carrot, pear, organic chicken, mung bean, buckwheat, jujube date

Remedies

1. Eat frequent, small meals and drink more liquids.

2. Juice and drink daily fresh water chestnut, lotus root, pear, watermelon and carrots.

3. Make soup from lotus seed, white fungus and figs.

4. Chop garlic finely and stir fry with egg white, parsley and diced yams.

5. Make soup from cabbage, azuki beans, winter melon and pumpkin.

6. Make chicken soup with garlic, onions, scallions, ginger and daikon radish. Drink soup or cook rice porridge with the broth.

7. Make buckwheat and rice porridge with chestnuts and longan fruit(Euphoria longan).

Avoid: dairy products, alcohol, coffee, sugar, fatty or fried foods, overly spicy foods, cold and raw foods, tomato, eggplant, bell pepper, shellfish

CHRONIC SINUSITIS

This condition is due to an acute inflammation of the nasal passages over a long period of time. There is often drainage or congestion, difficulty breathing through the nose, sometimes dryness of the nostrils, headaches, and ringing in the ears.

Recommendations: ginger, green onions, magnolia flower, bananas, garlic, black mushrooms, chrysanthemum flowers, mulberry leaves, apricot kernels. Get plenty of fresh air.

Remedies:
1. Make tea from magnolia flower, basil, ginger, and green onion; drink 3 times daily for at least 1 week.

2. Combine magnolia flowers and eggs, cook together and eat.

3. Make tea from mulberry leaves and chrysanthemums, then cook rice porridge in the tea, adding apricot kernels.

4. Mash green onions, soak cotton balls and alternately put in nostrils after having washed them with salt water.

5. Make garlic juice, add olive oil and soak cotton balls and alternately put in nostrils after having washed them with salt water.

6. Cook black mushrooms into a concentrated soup, then slowly use a dropper to put drops into the nose.

7. Boil tea of mint, basil, and ginger. While boiling the tea, inhale the steam through the nose, 3 times daily for at least 2 months.

Avoid: extremes of exposure to weather elements, coffee, smoking, stress, picking the nose, polluted air and smog

COMMON COLD

There are two basic types or stages of colds. In Chinese terminology they are the *wind cold type* and the *wind heat type*. They have different symptoms and different treatments.

1. WIND COLD TYPE
This type often occurs with a change in weather or when one is exposed to wind and cold. With a weak immune function these pathogens enter the skin. The symptoms could include chills, fever,. no sweating, headache, body ache, stiff neck, and clear copious nasal discharge. This is often the first stage of a cold. When the pathogens are at this initial,

superficial stage, we seek to sweat them out. A hot bath or dry sauna could be of benefit to start the sweating process.

Recommendations: ginger, garlic, mustard greens and seeds, grapefruit peel, cilantro, parsnip, scallions, cinnamon, basil, soupy rice porridge, and eating as little as possible so as not to burden the system with a lot of digestion.

Remedies:

1. Lightly boil for 5 minutes garlic, ginger, green onion, basil, mustard, or cinnamon, drink the tea; go to bed and prepare to sweat.

2. Drink cilantro and ginger tea.

3. Drink scallion and basil tea.

4. Make tea from dried grapefruit peel.

5. Make tea from mustard greens, cilantro and green onion.

6. Make tea from parsnip and ginger.

Avoid: shellfish, heavy proteins and fats, meats, all vinegars. Vinegar closes the pores and *traps the thief in the house.*

2. WIND HEAT TYPE

This type of common cold is characterized by high fever, some chills, sweating, sore throat, cough, headache, body ache, and yellow nasal discharge or sputum.

Recommendations: mint, cabbage, chrysanthemum flowers, burdock root, cilantro, dandelion, apples, pears, bitter melon, drink plenty of fluids, and get plenty of rest

Remedies:

1. Drink cabbage broth freely.

2. Drink cilantro and mint tea. 3. Drink mint, chrysanthemum and dandelion tea.

4. Drink mint, dandelion and licorice tea.

5. Drink burdock tea.

Avoid: shellfish, meats, vinegar, drafts, hot foods

CONSTIPATION

Constipation is a lack of regular evacuation of the bowels or difficulty in defecation. The resulting symptoms may include bloating, abdominal pain, abdominal hardness, and bad breath. We should evacuate at least once daily, with the optimal times energy-wise being from 5-7 A.M. The longer the waste remains in the intestines, the drier it gets and the more difficult to pass. Strained evacuation leads to hemorrhoids. Regular enemas or colonics are not a healthy solution to the problem. It is best to set a certain time for evacuation and train the body to respond accordingly. Rubbing the belly in a clockwise direction 100 times can stimulate the peristalsis of the intestines. Breathing with the mouth open is also beneficial in stimulating a bowel movement.

Recommendations: bananas, apples, walnuts, figs, spinach, peaches, pears, pine nuts, sesame seeds, mulberries, grapefruit, yams, honey, azuki (red) beans, apricot kernel, milk, yogurt, alfalfa sprouts, beets, cabbage, bok choy, cauliflower, potato, Chinese cabbage, salt water

Remedies:

1. Eat 2 bananas on an empty stomach, followed by a glass of water.

2. Drink a glass of lukewarm water with 2 teaspoons of honey on an empty stomach.

3. Drink blended beets and cabbage on an empty stomach.

4. Make beet soup.

5. Eat 5-10 figs on an empty stomach, followed by a glass of water.

6. Drink a glass of lukewarm water with 2 teaspoons of salt, on an empty stomach. This remedy should be used as a last resort when nothing else has worked and should not be used by those with edema or hypertension.

7. Eat a fresh apple on an empty stomach.

8. Drink mulberry juice.

9. Eat lightly steamed asparagus and cabbage at night before retiring.

Avoid: stress, tension, spicy foods, fried foods, meat

CORONARY HEART DISEASE

This is a condition in which the arteries that supply the heart become hardened and clogged, eventually leading to deprivation of oxygen and nourishment to the heart, thereby causing heart attack. Recent research has attributed the cause of coronary heart disease to faulty diet, obesity, continuous stress and tension, mental fatigue, hypertension, diabetes, low thyroid function, and smoking. Typical symptoms with coronary heart disease are dizziness, vertigo, palpitations, chest fullness, shortness of breath, pain in the chest area, irregular heart beat, spontaneous sweating, hardness in the lips and tongue, and angina pain when there is an obstruction.

Recommendations: American ginseng, brown rice, black fungus, sea cucumber, Chinese black dates, peanuts, vinegar, Shitake mushrooms, celery, seaweed, cassia seeds, lotus roots, jelly fish, chrysanthemums, hawthorn berries, water chestnuts, mung beans, pearl barley, peach kernels, ginger, soy sprouts, mung sprouts, other sprouts, wheat bran, buckwheat, persimmons, bananas, watermelon, sunflower seeds, lotus seeds, black sesames, wheat, garlic, green tea

Folk Remedies:

1. Take 3 grams American ginseng and cook with 1 c. brown rice and some rock sugar. Cook into a porridge and consume every morning.

2. Take black fungus and black mushrooms, soak overnight then steam 1 hour and eat before bedtime.

3. Take sea cucumber, Chinese black dates and steam together. Eat every morning on an empty stomach.

4. Soak 10 - 15 peanuts in rice vinegar for 24 hours and consume in the morning both the peanuts and the rice vinegar.

5. Cook tea from white or button mushrooms and Chinese black dates. Take 2 times daily for 1 month.

6. Make tea from seaweed, cassia seed, and lotus root; drink the tea and eat the seaweed and lotus root 2 times daily for at least 1 month.

7. Combine jellyfish, water chestnut, and rice vinegar; cook together into a soup.

8. Cook celery and yellow squash soup and eat once a day for at least 20 days.

9. Make tea from chrysanthemum flowers, hawthorn berries, and cassia seeds. Drink 1 c. 3 times daily for at least 20 days.

10. Take black fungus, pearl barley, and dried orange peel and boil into soup.

11. Grind betel nut and hawthorn berries; add rice flour, stir together and steam. Eat often.

12. Take 1 T. honey, 3 times a day.

13. Steam soy and alfalfa sprouts together and add some rice vinegar.

14. Slightly roast wheat and oat bran with black sesame and sunflower seeds. Sprinkle on vegetables or porridge.

15. Drink at least 2 c. green tea every day.

16. Go on a watermelon fast for 3 consecutive days.

17. Take peach kernel, safflowers, hawthorn berries, and make tea. Drink 2 c. daily for at least 1 month.

Avoid: fatty foods, stimulating foods, spicy foods, coffee, smoking, alcohol, simple carbohydrates (sugar, white flour), salt, stress, tension, worrying, emotional stimulation, lack of sleep

DIABETES

Diabetes is characterized by a high level of sugar in the blood and urine. Symptoms include excessive thirst, hunger, and urination. The Chinese refer to this condition as *exhaustion syndrome.* Proper exercise is of utmost importance in stimulating normal glandular functions; exercises such as T'ai Chi Ch'uan, Chi Gong, or the 8 Treasures are particularly valuable.

Recommendations: pumpkin, wheat, mung beans, winter melon, celery, pears, spinach, yams, peas, sweet rice, soybeans, tofu, mulberries, squash, daikon radish, cabbage, organic pig or chicken pancreas, peach, millet

Remedies:
1. Eat a slice of pumpkin with each meal.

2. Make pumpkin and yam pie with no sweeteners.

3. Prepare soup from cabbage, yam, winter melon, and lentils.

4. Drink daikon, celery, carrot, and spinach juice.

5. Steam tofu, cool to room temperature, add sesame oil and slices of raw squash.

6. Make soup from mung beans, peas, and barley.

7. Drink chrysanthemum tea whenever thirsty.

8. Eat non-sweetened sweet rice cake or mochi between meals.

9. Steam millet with yam and a few dates.

Avoid: sweets, sugar, honey, molasses, smoking, alcohol, caffeine, spicy foods, and most raw fruits

DIARRHEA

This is characterized by the frequent passage of abnormally watery stools, usually caused by increased peristalsis, irritation of the intestines through improper diet, drugs, bacterial infections, parasites, or worms. This differs from dysentery in that diarrhea is generally due to digestive weakness, biological imbalance, and in general is a chronic condition. Dysentery, on the other hand, is caused by an infectious condition.

Recommendations: garlic, black pepper, blueberries, cinnamon, raspberry leaves, lotus seeds, burned rice, yams, sweet potatoes, fresh fig leaves, peas, buckwheat, litchi, guava peel, apples, charcoaled bread, ginger, pearl barley, basil, unripe prunes

Remedies:

1. Cook rice porridge with lotus seed and yam or with barley.

2. Eat burnt rice or bread.

3. Make tea from dried litchi and Chinese black date.

4. Take 2 T. dried apples, 3 times daily on an empty stomach with warm water.

5. Cook rice porridge with ginger and black pepper.

6. Drink black tea.

7. Take 2 bulbs of garlic, baked until black. Then boil in water and drink the tea.

8. Make tea from guava peel.

9. Make tea from ginger, fennel, basil, and Chinese black dates.

10. Make tea from unripe prunes.

11. Take sweet rice porridge.

Avoid: cold, raw foods, most fruits, juices, overeating

DYSENTERY

Dysentery is a condition of intestinal inflammation characterized by abdominal pain, intense, urgent, watery diarrhea with foul smelling, bloody or mucus feces, dry mouth, thirst, and decreased urination. To prevent dehydration, plenty of fluids should be consumed. The person will sometimes defecate 30 or 40 times daily. Food poisoning can be a possible cause. Dysentery is considered to be contagious, usually transmitted through unsanitary food or water. Sometimes the person also has vomiting.

Recommendations: buckwheat, sweet potatoes, peas, celery, scallions, taro root, ginger, garlic, carrots, daikon radish, green pepper, winter melon, cantaloupe, bitter melon, hawthorn berries, figs, Chinese prunes, pears, persimmons, guavas, olives, sunflower seeds, lotus roots, tea, soy products, corn, pumpkins, water chestnuts, squash, honey, mung beans, cherries, pineapples, watermelon, brown rice, oats, chicken eggs (only if chronic)

Remedies:

1. Take carrot juice mixed with a little ginger juice, honey, and green tea; drink 1 cup daily.

2. Make mung bean soup and drink throughout the day.

3. Take ginger, garlic, celery, and peas stir fried together; incorporate into regular diet.

4. Eat 4 persimmons daily.

5. Soak Chinese prunes in rice wine for 3 days; take 10 prunes 2 times daily.

6. Make sweet potato and pumpkin mush and have 3 times a day, for breakfast, lunch, and dinner.

7. Steam black fungus with a little sugar in about 1 1/2 cups of water.

8. Charcoal dried ginger, powder it, and take 1 teaspoon with soupy rice.

9. Drink sour prune tea before meals on an empty stomach.

10. Drink plum peel tea.

11. Cook brown rice with persimmon *cap* and consume the rice.

12. Consume eggs that are cooked with rice vinegar. This remedy is only appropriate for chronic cases of dysentery.

Avoid: dairy products, high-fiber foods, hard to digest foods, fried foods, meats, fish, raw foods, cold foods, chicken eggs (in acute cases of dysentery)

ECZEMA

This is a common skin condition that often affects extremities, genitalia, as well as other parts. The skin lesion is characterized by a raised spot that turns into a blister and eventually erupts, ulcerates and then forms a scab which is later sloughed off. It can cause extreme itching and pain.

Recommendations: potatoes, broccoli, dandelion, mung bean, seaweed, pearl barley, azuki beans, cornsilk, water chestnut, winter melon, watermelon

Remedies:

1. Mash fresh potato and apply locally, changing every 4 hours, for 3 days.

2. Apply honey to area.

3. Apply mashed daikon radish to area.

4. Internally, make tea from mung beans and pearl barley.

5. Make tea from dandelion and cornsilk.

6. Make tea from azuki beans, pearl barley, and cornsilk. Drink tea and eat the solids 3 times daily.

7. Boil soup from seaweed and winter melon, drinking at least once a day for 10 days.

8. Externally, wash with equal portions of salt and borax, dissolved in warm water; wash area 2 - 3 times daily.

9. Make tea from lily bulbs, Chinese black dates, and mulberries, drink 3 times daily for at least 10 days.

Avoid: external stimulation such as extreme weather condition of wind, cold, dampness, dryness, heat; excessive sun exposure, chemical exposure, soap (use clean water to bath)

EDEMA/SWELLING

Edema is a condition of swelling due to abnormal accumulation of fluids in the cells. It can occur any place in the body, however, the common places that edema occurs are face, lower extremities, and abdomen. Abdominal edema can cause ascites and is usually related to liver dysfunction such as cirrhosis of the liver. The treatment chosen is to promote diuresis and ease urination. Heart, kidney, and lungs are the organs that may be involved.

Recommendations: red (azuki) beans, corn, ginger skin, winter melon, winter melon skin, squash, apples, mulberries, peaches, tangerines, coconuts, seaweeds, fish, celery, green onions, garlic, bamboo shoots, spinach, water chestnuts, millet, wheat, black beans, pearl barley, carrots, watermelon, oats, beef

Remedies:
1. Take fish, preferably carp, and cook into soup with azuki beans.

Use 10 cups of water and cook down to 1 cup; consume only the liquid.

2. Take winter melon rind and azuki bean and enough water to cover; cook and eat 3 times daily.

3. Drink blended juice of apple, carrot, and green onion 2 times daily.

4. Boil tea from ginger skin.

5. Cook together pearl barley, mung beans, and azuki beans into a soup; consume 3 times daily. You may also add black beans to this soup.

6. Daily diet should be on the bland side, including plenty of vegetables and fish.

7. Eat plenty of watermelon, if it is summertime.

8. Drink coconut juice daily.

9. Cook oats and mung beans to a mush and consume until swelling subsides.

10. Consume soupy pearl barley.

11. Drink beef stew broth.

12. Drink tea made from watermelon rind.

Avoid: rich foods, salty foods, lamb, stimulating foods, wine, garlic, pepper, shellfish, fatty foods, greasy foods

GLAUCOMA

This is an eye disease characterized by an increase in the pressure inside of the eyes. Its onset can be either acute or chronic. The sufferer often complains that lights have halos around them. The condition can progress to a point in which the pressure causes atrophy of the optic nerve, leading to blindness. During the onset there may be pain, headaches, nausea, vomiting, and blurry vision.

Recommendations: chrysanthemum, mint, oyster shells, mulberries, black sesame, betel nuts, lycii fruit, cassia seeds, grapefruit, lemons, oranges, carrots, beets, beet tops

Remedies:
1. Boil tea from mulberries, oyster shell, and black sesame, drink 3 times daily.

2. Make tea from chrysanthemum and mint, drink 2 times daily.

3. Boil tea from betel nut, drink 2 times daily.

4. Boil tea from cassia seeds, orange peels, beets, and lycii fruit, then use the tea to cook rice porridge; add a little honey.

Avoid: Self treatment is not usually recommended due to the seriousness of this condition. Seek professional guidance for close observation of the condition. Avoid visual stimulation, stimulating foods, alcohol, drugs, smoking, coffee, salt, drinking too much water.

HEADACHE

There are many different types of headaches, such as migraines, ones caused by muscular tension, hypertension, common cold, mental stress, hormonal changes, and eye strain. Each type of headache would have a corresponding treatment.

Recommendations: chrysanthemum flowers, mint, green onions, ginger, oyster shells, pearl barley, carrots, prunes, buckwheat, peach kernels

Remedies:
FOR HEADACHES DUE TO COMMON COLD OR FLU:
1. Make tea from ginger and green onions, boiling for 5 minutes; drink and try to sweat.

2. Steam aching portion of head over mint and cinnamon tea that is cooking, then dry head afterwards, avoiding catching a draft.

3. Make tea from chrysanthemum flowers, cassia seeds and drink.

4. Make buckwheat meal into a paste and apply to painful area until it sweats.

5. Drink green tea.

6. Make rice porridge and add garlic and green onions. Eat while hot, then get under covers and sweat.

FOR HEADACHES DUE TO HIGH BLOOD PRES-
SURE, MENSTRUAL CYCLES, EMOTIONAL STRESS
OR TENSION, OR MIGRAINES:

1. Make carrot juice. If headache is on left side, squirt carrot juice into left nostril; if on right side, squirt into right nostril; if both sides are painful, squirt into both nostrils.

2. Take lemon juice and 1/2 T. baking soda mixed in a glass of water and drink.

3. Make tea of Chinese prunes, mint, and green tea.

4. Make tea of oyster shells and chrysanthemum flowers, slowly boiling the shells for 1 1/2 hours, then adding the flowers for the last 30 minutes.

5. Mash peach kernels and walnuts, mix with rice wine and lightly roast it; take 2 T. three times daily.

6. Rinse head with warm water, gradually increasing the temperature to hot.

Avoid: spicy food, lack of sleep, alcohol, smoking, excess stimulation, eye strain, stress.

Menstrual type headaches usually are accompanied by Premenstrual Syndrome (P.M.S.). Please refer to that section for further details.

HEMORRHOIDS

This is a common condition in America today, related to constipation. With dry stools the person strains to move the bowels and causes friction with the rectal tissues. Sometimes it can cause bleeding. Hemorrhoids can be due to over consumption of alcohol, spicy or fried foods; lack of exercise; sitting or standing for too long; too much sex; pregnancy; or chronic constipation. A hemorrhoid is a varicose vein in the rectum and can be very painful.

Recommendations: sea cucumber, black fungus, water chestnut, buckwheat, tangerines, figs, plums, fish, prunes, guavas, bamboo shoots, mung beans, winter melon, black sesame seeds, persimmons, bananas, squash, cucumbers, taro, tofu, cooling foods

Remedies:

1. Soak lower body in a warm bath to which has been added the tea of either mugwort (Artemisia argyi), carrot tops, or figs. Bath should be warm enough to induce sweating and done daily.

2. Take black fungus with rice every morning for breakfast on an empty stomach; do this for 1 month.

3. Steam sea cucumber without salt or spices and eat for immediate pain relief.

4. Roast and grind black sesame seeds, take with warm water and honey every night before retiring.

5. Steam dried persimmons and eat.

6. Wash hemorrhoid with winter melon tea.

7. Boil papaya tea for 2 hours, without the skin, and soak area.

8. Grind mung bean powder, boil with dandelion greens and wash area with the tea.

9. Steam figs, add honey and steam again several times, until it becomes soggy; consume every day.

10. Insert a raw potato suppository after each bowel movement.

11. Eat a banana everyday on an empty stomach.

FOR BLEEDING HEMORRHOIDS, THE FOLLOWING REMEDIES CAN BE USED:

1. Take black fungus cooked with brown sugar; consume daily.

2. Every morning on an empty stomach, eat 3 bananas with some honey.

3. Before breakfast and after dinner every day for 2 weeks, eat a fresh squash.

4. Make taro root soup and eat regularly until bleeding stops and hemorrhoid heals.

5. Mash fresh plums and take with lukewarm water 3 times daily.

6. Wash area with hot water, then apply a cotton ball that has been soaked in garlic juice. Change cotton every hour.

Avoid: stimulating foods, spicy foods, alcohol, smoking, constipation, stress, lack of exercise, standing or sitting too long

HEPATITIS

Hepatitis is a liver condition that can be caused by many drugs and toxic agents, as well as by numerous viruses. The manifestations include jaundice, anorexia, nausea, vomiting, malaise, fever, tender liver area, and flu-like symptoms. Upon examination of the blood, the liver enzymes are abnormally high. Viral Hepatitis A is generally transmitted via the fecal-oral route, whereas viral Hepatitis B is transmitted via blood and sexual fluids. Bed rest is necessary in the initial stages. Hepatitis can also become a chronic case.

Recommendations: rice, barley, millet, azuki bean, pearl barley, squash, cucumber, grapefruit, Ling Zhi mushroom, corn silk, dandelion greens, beet greens, pears, water chestnut, carrot, cabbage, spinach, celery, winter melon, rice vinegar, apple, orange, pineapple, lotus root, watermelon

Remedies:
1. Cook lotus root and puree, then cook into rice or millet porridge.

2. Make tea from corn silk, dandelion and beet greens. Drink regularly as a beverage.

3. Juice watermelon, celery and pears.

4. Make mung bean soup with pearl barley.

5. Soak grapefruit and peel in rice vinegar overnight, then take 1 teaspoon in 1 cup of warm liquid.

6. Make tea from Ling Zhi and jujube dates.

7. Take cucumber juice on empty stomach every morning.

8. Charcoal grapefruit peel and take 1/2 teaspoon with rice water after every meal.

9. Make soup from winter melon and kobocha squash.

Avoid: dairy products, alcohol, coffee, sugar, fatty and fried foods, overly spicy foods, cold and raw foods, tomato, eggplant, bell peppers, shellfish.

HIVES

Hives is a skin condition which is characterized by an intermittent attack of extreme itching which results in welts, mostly on the arms, legs, back, and face. These elevated spots can spread throughout the entire body with scratching. It may be brought on by an exposure to an allergen or after consumption of shellfish. This condition in Chinese Medicine is considered invasion of *wind*.

Recommendations: winter melon rind, chrysanthemum,vinegar, papaya, ginger, Chinese black dates, dried prunes, black sesame, black beans, litchi, pearl barley, cornsilk, soybeans, mung beans, licorice, hawthorn berries, peach kernels, maple leaves, Shitake mushrooms, mint

Remedies:

1. Externally, take a sea salt bath, and rub salt on the hives.

2. Boil a thick tea from fresh maple leaves for an external wash of hives.

3. Internally, drink tea made from 15 g. gypsum, 9 g. hawthorn berries, 60 g. black beans, some winter melon rind and chrysanthemum flowers. Add some honey and drink 3 times daily. 4. Cook together papaya, ginger, and rice vinegar until vinegar is dried up. Eat the ginger and papaya 2 times daily for at least 10 days.

5. Mix honey with rice wine and steam. Drink 2 T. on an empty stomach every morning.

6. Cook together black sesame, black bean, and Chinese black dates and eat at least once daily.

7. Make tea of dried litchi, add some brown sugar and take 3 times daily.

8. Make tea of lotus seeds and 1/2 t. pearl powder.

9. Make tea of cornsilk and pearl barley and drink 2 times daily for at least 10 days.

10. Take equal portions of mung and soy beans, grind into powder, add water and boil 15 minutes. Then strain and drink 1 c. 2 times daily.

11. Make tea of licorice, mung beans, and gypsum; drink 3 times daily for at least 3 days.

12. Eat 2 - 3 dried prunes daily.

Avoid: shellfish, allergic foods

HYPERTENSION

Hypertension, or high blood pressure, is characterized by a wiry and rapid pulse, headache, dizziness, tinnitus, blurry vision, palpitations, chest tightness or fullness, fatigue, insomnia, vertigo, and numbness of the extremities. It is commonly caused by hardening of the arteries, kidney dysfunction, or liver dysfunction. The normal range of blood pressure is between 70 - 85 mm Hg for diastolic and 100 - 135 mm Hg for systolic measurement.

Recommendations: celery, spinach, garlic, bananas, sunflower seeds, honey, tofu, mung beans, bamboo shoots, seaweed, vinegar, tomatoes, water chestnuts, corn, apples, persimmons, peas, buckwheat, jellyfish, watermelon, hawthorn berries, eggplant, plums, mushrooms, lemons, lotus root, chrysanthemum, cassia seeds

Remedies:

1. Drink warm celery juice 3 times daily.

2. Eat 2 raw tomatoes on an empty stomach every day for a month.

3. Drink water, vinegar and honey regularly.

4. Drink chrysanthemum and spinach tea regularly.

5. Drink cornsilk tea.

6. Sleep on a pillow of chrysanthemum flowers to draw the heat out of the head.

7. Make mung bean soup.

8. Take garlic oil capsules to clean out the arteries. The capsules have the advantage of not overly stimulating the taste buds in the warming direction. The taste buds start the functions of many physiological processes; the spicy flavor can be too stimulating, in general, for hypertensive individuals.

9. Steam or bake jellyfish about 12 minutes, add vinegar, soy sauce, and sesame oil; take daily for about 2 months.

10. Steam tofu, cool to room temperature, add vinegar and sesame oil. This can be combined with soupy rice for a nutritious breakfast.

11. Make lotus root tea and drink 3 c. daily for one month.

12. Make tea from chrysanthemum flowers and cassia seeds and drink daily.

13. Steam white fungus for 2 hours and take before bed time.

14. Drink hawthorn berry tea continuously for a long period of time.

15. Make soup from abalone and seaweed.

16. During the summer months, make watermelon juice or eat watermelon every day.

17. Make tea from watermelon rind, mugwort, and mulberry branches, drink 3 c. daily for 2 months.

18. Take celery, white onion (sweet), garlic, water chestnuts, and tomatoes and 4 c. water; boil down to 1 c. and drink every night before bed.

19. Take seaweed, pearl barley and a little honey and cook into soup; eat every day for 5 days.

20. Mix pig bile and mung bean powder; take 1 t. twice daily for at least 8 days.

21. Take black or white mushrooms and cook soup daily.

22. Eat 3 apples daily.

23. Drink organic banana peel tea.

24. Make tea from one peeled lemon, 10 fresh water chestnuts, and 2 1/2 c. water.

25. Drink 3 glasses daily of unripened persimmon juice for 1 week.

Avoid: smoking, alcohol, spicy foods, coffee, caffeine, all stimulants, fatty or fried foods, salty foods, stress, constipation, potatoes, strong emotions, pork, overeating, and low levels of calcium* in the body.

For low calcium levels make tea from shells (oyster, abalone, mother of pearl) or fossils (dragon bones and teeth); strain and drink.

HYPOGLYCEMIA

This is a very common condition in America due to the stressful lifestyle and heavy sugar laden diet. Hypoglycemia is characterized by low blood sugar, chronic fatigue, nervousness, shakiness, headaches, fatigue when hungry, irritability or faintness if meal is late, sweet craving, waking at night hungry, night sweats, light-headedness, mood swings, depression, and difficulty concentrating.

Recommendations: sweet rice, brown rice, yams, potatoes, walnuts, tofu, soybeans, corn, fish, chicken, vegetables, black beans, nuts (a good snack between meals), mild exercise, regular meal schedule, 4-5 small meals daily

Avoid: simple carbohydrates such as white flour and sugar, honey, fructose, maple syrup, sweet fruits (eat very sparingly), coffee, smoking, fatty foods, fried foods, all stimulants

IMPOTENCE

This is a weak condition, most likely due to a nervous weakness, excessive stress, worrying, tension, physical fatigue, frequent masturbation, or excessive indulgence in sex. Impotence is characterized by not being able to have an erection when there is a desire to have intercourse, and there may be premature ejaculation. Other symptoms may include dizziness, insomnia, excessive dreams, low appetite, back pain, lower extremities weakness, knee pain, and fatigue.

Recommendations: scallions, scallion seeds, lamb, sea cucumber, shrimps, rooster, bitter melon seeds, ginseng, black beans, kidney beans, yams, lycii fruit, maintaining a calm composure. Tonifying foods are needed, thus, many of the remedies include meat, however, it does not have to be treated with meat.

Remedies:

1. Make lamb stew with daikon radish and Chinese black dates. Drink the broth and eat the lamb.

2. Make cake from black sweet rice, black sesame, black fungus, lotus seeds, walnuts, and black beans. Eat with 1/2 glass of red wine.

3. Steam a rooster with ginger.

4. Take dried shrimps, sea cucumber, and fennel, and dry roast and grind into a powder and take 1 t. 3 times daily with rice wine.

5. Roast and grind bitter melon seeds, take 1 t. 3 times daily with rice wine.

6. Make tea from walnuts, lotus seeds, pearl barley, Chinese black dates, and lycii fruit, and drink 3 times daily.

7. Take 50 grams of chopped ginseng and 1/2 bottle of white liquor (like vodka or gin), seal bottle, shake bottle daily and preserve for 1 month. Drink 1 shot every night with dinner for at least 20 days.

8. Cook together scallions, shrimp, and egg and take with a shot of white liquor.

Avoid: obscene visual stimulation, dairy products, sweets, masturbation, overwork, too much sex

INDIGESTION

This is a condition of poor digestion due to weak stomach, lack of digestive enzymes, or eating too fast. This causes a stagnation of food in the stomach, resulting in abdominal fullness or distention, bloating, and sometimes diarrhea due to insufficient digestion.

Recommendations: hawthorn berries, papayas, sweet potatoes or

yams, figs, pineapples, brown rice, oats, pearl barley, sweet rice, daikon radish, black sesame seeds, apples, oranges. It is important to eat slowly and chew the food properly; digestion begins in the mouth.

Remedies:

1. Dry and age orange peel for about 1 month. Boil tea and take after meals or simply suck on the peel for indigestion.

2. Eat papaya 2 times daily, in any form.

3. Eat sweet potato cooked with brown sugar and water. In the last 3 minutes of cooking this mush, add some rice wine. Eat regularly for 2 weeks to improve digestion.

4. Blend daikon radish juice and take after meals.

5. Roast black sesame seeds with salt and take with warm water.

6. Eat a leaf of fresh mugwort, or blend into a juice.

7. Take apple, lemon, or orange juice after meals; or eat an apple after each meal.

8. Consume 1/2 c. of overdone rice (from bottom of pan) mixed with cardamon, fennel and orange peels.

9. Make tea from sweet rice sprouts and malt.

Avoid: rich foods, fatty foods, tension and stress while eating, reading the newspaper or watching television while eating as this takes energy away from digestion.

KIDNEY WEAKNESS

This is a common ailment among Americans, characterized by weakness and lack of energy. In Chinese medicine the Kidney system involves much more than just filtering water. It also includes storing the essence of life (sperms and eggs); controlling the bones, bone marrow and the brain (called *the sea of marrow)*; growth, maintenance, and reproduction; producing blood; and opening to the ear. The adrenal function is included in the Kidney system; thus adrenal exhaustion is Kidney exhaustion. Weakness of the Kidneys often manifests as problems in the back, knees, ears, or reproductive functions. The Kidney is of great importance to health and longevity. Kidney function (and resulting problems) can be divided into Kidney Yang and Kidney Yin.

1. KIDNEY YANG DEFICIENCY

This is characterized by impotence, infertility, coldness, swollen extremities, swollen face, frequent urination, premature ejaculation, diarrhea, low sexual drive, low energy, fatigue, pale face and tongue, low back pain, knee pain or weakness, deafness, ringing in the ears, and a general feeling as though the *fire of life is about out.*

Recommendations: warming foods, chicken, lamb, scallions, sesame seeds, fish, baked tofu, soybeans, walnuts, eggs, lentils, black beans, lotus seeds, a little wine, ginger, cinnamon bark tea

Avoid: cold foods, cold fruits, raw foods

2. KIDNEY YIN DEFICIENCY

In this condition there is not enough water to cool the fire so it manifests as heat symptoms. These may include irritability, insomnia, red cheeks, night sweats, low afternoon fever, damp palms, damp soles of the feet, dry mouth, low back pain, seminal emissions, ear ringing, red tongue, and blurry vision. 95% of the time Kidney Yin deficiency occurs in thin people since Yin corresponds to substance.

Recommendations: cooling foods, mulberries, apples, peaches, pears, fresh vegetables, mung bean, most beans, soybeans, tofu, soy sprouts, chrysanthemum flowers

Avoid: hot foods, spicy foods, smoking, alcohol, stress, and strong emotions

MASTITIS

This is an inflammation of the mammary glands, often occurring 3 - 4 weeks after delivery. It is a very common condition, resulting from an obstructed mammary duct and accompanied by a bacterial infection. There may be distention of the breast, pain, swelling, redness on the surface, and fever. As the condition progresses, the symptoms may worsen and the patient may have chills, fever, increase in white blood cell count, swollen and painful lymph glands in the armpits, pus and ulceration of breast.

Recommendations: cooling foods such as cabbage, cucumber, dandelion, lettuce, malt, reed root, lotus root, honeysuckle. It is important to keep the affected breast clean.

Remedies:
1. Make tea from malt (sprouted oat), drink 3 times daily.
2. Externally, take egg white mixed with green onions and apply to the area, changing 2 - 3 times daily.

3. Make tea from dandelion and honey, drink 3 times daily for at least 5 days.

4. Make tea from honeysuckle, mint, and licorice, drink tea and apply the solids locally.

5. Boil dandelions into tea then condense into a syrup and add to rice porridge. Eat 3 times daily for 5 days.

6. Combine cabbage, lettuce, and dandelions to make a poultice for external application.

Avoid: spicy, stimulating foods, coffee, smoking, alcohol, dairy products (especially if there is pus), breast feeding

MENOPAUSE

This is the time when a woman stops menstruating completely, usually occurring between 45 and 50 years of age. It may occur slowly or suddenly. Symptoms may include hot flashes, weakness, depression, emotional instability, anxiety, lack of concentration, irritability, headaches, insomnia, night sweats, and dryness.

Recommendations: black beans, sesame seeds, soybeans, walnuts, lycii berries, mulberries, yams, licorice, Chinese black dates, lotus seeds, chrysanthemum flowers. Try to remain calm.

Remedies:

1. Cook black beans with rice into porridge, eat 2 times daily.

2. Roast sesame seeds and add to rice porridge for breakfast.

3. Steam chicken with lycii berries and yam.

4. Make tea from chrysanthemum and cassia seeds and take 3 times daily.

5. Take walnuts, lotus seeds, and sunflower seeds and make a porridge with rice.

6. Stew millet, mulberries, lamb, and lycii fruit.

7. Make tea from licorice, Chinese black dates, and wheat. This will help extreme mood swings and depression.

Avoid: stress, tension, stimulants

MORNING SICKNESS

This is characterized by nausea and vomiting and affects some women during the first few months of pregnancy, usually clearing up after the third month. It occurs particularly in the morning, although in serious cases, it may last all day. Accompanying symptoms may include headache, dizziness, and exhaustion. One should seek treatment right away as it will affect nourishment to the fetus.

Recommendations: lentils, grapefruit peel, carp, ginger, orange peel, bamboo shavings, persimmon *cap*, millet

Remedies:

1. Grind lentils into powder then take 2 T. with rice porridge, 3 times daily.

2. Make tea from ginger and grapefruit peel, drink 3 times daily.

3. Steam carp with ginger and cardamon for 30 minutes. Eat daily for at least 1 week.

4. Make tea from ginger, orange peels, and a little bit of brown sugar.

5. Take the *cap* off the persimmon, make tea and drink 3 times daily.

6. Make fresh scallion juice and fresh ginger juice and add a little bit of sweetener. Take 2 - 3 t. 3 times daily.

As soon as the morning sickness stops, discontinue the remedies.

Avoid: overeating, heavy meats

MOUTH SORES (ULCERS)

This condition includes herpes simplex, fever blisters and canker sores. It is basically an ulceration on or in the mouth. One may also experience pain, hot sensation, irritability, insomnia, headache, dizziness, palpitations, and bad breath.

Recommendations: mung beans, daikon, carrots, lotus root, persimmon *caps*, mint, honeysuckle flower

Remedies:

1. Make juice from carrots and lotus root and rinse the mouth 3 - 4 times a day for at least 4 days.

2. Take 5 - 6 persimmon *caps* and boil tea. When cool, rinse mouth 4 - 5 times a day.

3. Apply honey to local area to help heal faster.

4. Char eggplant into ashes, powder and mix with honey. Apply to the sores. 5. Boil mung beans soup and eat on an empty stomach.

6. Grind mung beans into powder, mix with honey; apply to area.

7. Rub sea salt on the sores, 3 times a day for 2 days. Also rinse mouth with salt water.

Avoid: spicy foods, stimulating foods, smoking, stress, alcohol, coffee, chocolate, constipation

NEPHRITIS (ACUTE)

This is an acute kidney infection. This condition is characterized by some type of infection that precedes the condition, such as laryngitis, tonsillitis, scarlet fever, or mumps. There may be swelling beginning in the face area then spreading throughout the body in about 2 days, followed by blood in the urine, hypertension, headache, dizziness, fatigue, malaise, low appetite, nausea, vomiting, and scanty urination.

Recommendations: black beans, mung beans, azuki beans, pearl barley, garlic, carp, winter melon, watermelon, watermelon rind, reed root, cornsilk, sweet rice, lotus root, water chestnuts

Remedies:

1. Cook soup with azuki beans, winter melon rind, water melon rind and cornsilk. Drink at least 3 - 4 times daily.

2. Make tea from lotus root, drink 4 large glasses daily.

3. Do a watermelon fast or eat lots of watermelon.

4. Cook soup with carp, azuki beans, winter melon, and green onions. Start with 5 c. water and cook down to 3 c. Drink the soup and sweat.

5. Make tea from cornsilk, cooking for 1 hour, then strain and cook again until almost dry, then add some fructose powder. Then take 1 T. 3 times daily dissolved in warm water.

6. Cook rice porridge with pearl barley, black bean and water chestnuts.

7. Make juice from carrots, celery, cucumbers, and squash.

Avoid: stimulating (sour, spicy, salty) foods, alcohol, caffeine, smoking, overworking, high protein foods

NEPHRITIS (CHRONIC)

This can result from acute nephritis that is not properly treated; or, a low immunity, causing kidney infection. The symptoms include swelling, hypertension, hyperprotein urea, fatigue, headache, dizziness, and achiness. If this condition does not get proper treatment, over a period of time it can cause damage to the kidney, leading to uremia.

Recommendations: ginger, Chinese black dates, sweet rice, soybeans, winter melon, carp, yams, mung beans, black beans

Remedies:

1. Make rice porridge and add ginger, cinnamon, and Chinese black dates; eat for breakfast and dinner.

2. Remove the internal organs of a duck and stuff it with 4 - 5 cloves of garlic, then cook in soup. Do not add salt. Drink the broth and eat the duck every other day.

3. Cook carp with soy beans, winter melon, and green onions into soup. Eat once a day for at least 20 days.

4. Cook rice porridge with yams and eat for breakfast and dinner.

5. Steam together crab, garlic, and white wine, and eat once daily for 15 days.

6. Boil tea from cornsilk, winter melon rind, watermelon rind, and azuki beans.

7. Crush entire watermelon (with rind) and slowly cook to a thick syrup. Take 2 T. syrup in warm water 3 times daily.

Avoid: stimulating (sour, spicy, salty) foods, alcohol, caffeine, smoking, overworking, high protein foods

PREMENSTRUAL SYNDROME (P.M.S.)

P.M.S. is a condition that occurs after ovulation or before menstruation, due to hormonal fluctuations. It may be characterized by abdominal cramps, bloating, backache, headache, tension, irritability, low energy, and mood swings. A healthy woman should have little or no discomfort during this time, however, approximately 70% of American women suffer from these symptoms. This is partially due to the large consumption of cold foods and drinks in this country that in turn cause the blood to stagnate. In Chinese terminology, P.M.S. is a condition of disharmony in the blood: either stagnant blood, not enough blood, or heat in the blood; and stagnation of Chi. Acupuncture, acupressure, herbs, diet, and Chi (Qi) Gong exercises are all very beneficial for relieving the symptoms and correcting the disharmony.

Recommendations: At least one week prior to the usual onset time of P.M.S. symptoms, consume some of the following: ginger, green onions, fennel, orange peel, spinach, walnuts, hawthorn berries, cinnamon, and black pepper, Chinese date, Dang Gui(Angelica sinensis)

Remedies:
1. Make tea from ginger, green onions, fennel, black pepper,

and orange peel, boiling for 10 minutes. Drink 3 times daily, starting at least 1 week before usual onset of P.M.S. symptoms. (Especially for those who feel cold.)

2. Make spinach soup, boiling for 30 minutes.

3. Make hawthorn berry and cinnamon tea.

4. See a Chinese Herbalist/Acupuncturist for herb formula.

Avoid: cold foods, raw foods, excessive consumption of fruit, vinegar, all shellfish, coffee, stimulants, sugar, dairy products, and smoking.

PROSTATE ENLARGEMENT

This condition generally effects older men (over 40). As the man ages the prostate can become swollen and the urethra and bladder become less elastic. Thus, symptoms usually include difficulty urinating, weak stream or dribbling.

Recommendations: pumpkin seeds, anise, tangerines, cherries, figs, litchis, sunflower seeds, mangos, seaweeds

Remedies:

1. Roast pumpkin seeds or boil into tea and incorporate into the diet, 1 large handful 2 times daily.

2. Make tea from rhubarb root, peach kernels, winter melon seeds, pearl barley, azuki beans, and cornsilk; drink 3 times daily.

3. Boil fig tea.

Avoid: dairy products, rich foods, fatty foods, all stimulants such as alcohol, caffeine, and smoking; stress, tension, sex, and eating meat late in the day

PSORIASIS

This is a common skin condition, usually genetically inherited, characterized by pink or dull red lesions with silvery scaling. The skin may become very rough and scaly and may temporarily improve, although it is usually a chronic type of condition. When the scaling takes place one can also see reddish dots under the skin, accompanied by various degrees of itching and discomfort. It can affect any part of the body, and is usually worse during the winter time. In Western medicine, there is presently no treatment for psoriasis.

Recommendations: Chinese prunes, guava skins, pearl barley, vinegar, garlic, walnuts, cucumber, beet tops, dandelions, squash, mung beans

Remedies:
1. Take 15 peeled and sliced water chestnuts and 1 c. vinegar (preferably aged rice vinegar), slowly simmer in a non-metal pot for 20 minutes until water chestnuts absorb most of the vinegar. Then mash into a paste and seal in a jar. Spread evenly on a gauze pad and apply to affected area, changing daily if not too serious, 3 times daily if serious condition. Mild cases should show improvement within 5 days; serious conditions may take 2 weeks.

2. Take dried Chinese prunes, remove pits, and simmer into a tea, then condense into a syrup. Take 2 T. in warm water, 3 times daily.

3. Take peel from guava, char and powder it, mix with sesame oil into a paste and apply 2 times daily for 1 week.

4. Apply mashed garlic to the affected area, changing 2 times daily for 1 week.

5. Make porridge from lily bulb, gypsum, and rice. Eat once daily for at least 10 days.

6. Take mashed walnuts, use cotton to absorb the oil, apply the pulp 3 times daily.

Avoid: spicy food, stimulating food, alcohol, caffeine, smoking, excessive sun exposure

SEMINAL EMISSION (SPERMATORRHEA)

There are 2 types of this condition. The first type happens when one has a dream and then ejaculates during sleep, also known as a wet dream. The other type is when one has ejaculation without a dream, either during sleep or during waking hours. One may also have dizziness, back pain, leg pain, weakness, palpitations, shortness of breath, lethargy, or fatigue. These symptoms point to a weakness which if not dealt with can lead to degeneration.

Recommendations: lotus seeds, sea cucumber, yams, dried ginger, scallions, pearl barley, black beans, shrimps, seaweeds, cool showers daily

Remedies:
1. Steam scallions with shrimp and rice wine. Eat daily for at least 15 days or until condition improves.

2. Cook soup from sea cucumber, seaweed, and black beans. One can add walnuts also.

3. Cook sea cucumber with rice porridge and eat for breakfast every morning.

4. Cook pearl barley, black beans, walnuts, and scallions to make a porridge; eat every morning for breakfast.

5. Make tea from ginseng, Chinese black dates, and lotus seeds. Drink 3 times daily.

Avoid: spicy foods, stimulating foods, overworking, obscene visual images, masturbation, sleeping on one's back (sleep on the side instead)

SORE THROAT (LARYNGITIS)

Sore throat can be caused by various factors including common cold, flu, or eating too much spicy food. There may also be a lot of mucus, fever and chills, headaches, and so on.

Recommendations: carrots, olives, daikon, celery, seaweed, licorice, Chinese prunes, cilantro, mint. Drink a lot of water, and gargle with warm salt water.

Remedies:

1. Make tea from carrots and olives; drink 3 times daily for at least 1 week.

2. Make tea from daikon radish and green apples; drink 2 times daily.

3. Lightly cook seaweed, preserve with brown sugar for 3 days; eat daily for 1 week.

4. Make tea from cilantro, 1 T. green tea and a little salt, steeping for about 5 minutes.

5. Slowly chew and swallow rock sugar and cilantro.

6. For dry, hot throat, take a spoonful of honey in a glass of warm water, and drink.

Avoid: alcohol, smoking, pollution, sleeping with the mouth open, stimulating or spicy foods, fatty foods

STONES (GALL BLADDER, KIDNEY OR URINARY TRACT)

Various combinations of minerals can calcify or crystalize in the gallbladder, kidney, or urinary tract. These can range from the size of a grain of sand to 2 inches in diameter. Gallstones are a combination of bile and minerals and are characterized by pain in the right upper abdomen or pain in the corresponding area of the back and shooting up to the shoulder blade. Gallstones may also cause poor digestion of fats. If the gallstones obstruct the flow of bile, the result may be jaundice. Kidney stones are formed as the kidneys filter excessive minerals in an acid environment which combine with either excessive calcium or wastes in the blood. These are very painful, with the pain being in the kidney area of the lower back or the corresponding area on the front of the abdomen. There may also be painful or blocked urination with kidney stones.

Recommendations: cornsilk, water chestnuts, seaweed, beet tops, watermelon, celery, watercress, winter melon, pearl barley, walnuts, watermelon rind, winter melon rind, green tea powder, distilled water

Remedies:

1. Drink watermelon juice.

2. Drink celery, carrot, and water chestnut juice.

3. Drink cornsilk tea for water; 3-5 glasses daily.

4. Drink tea from beet tops, winter melon rind, and watermelon rind.

5. Take 2 teaspoons ground walnuts in cornsilk tea.

6. Take 1 teaspoon green tea powder in warm water 3 times daily.

After consuming any of the above diuretic remedies, do some mild jumping exercise to help break up the stones.

Avoid: spicy foods, fried foods, oily foods, coffee, hard water, spinach, citrus, tomatoes, spinach combined with tofu or dairy products

TINNITUS (EAR RINGING)

This is a common problem that has two major causes. The first is a local problem in which there may be a local obstruction or infection, nerve damage, or drug interference. The second stems more from a systemic condition such as coronary heart disease, hypertension, or kidney weakness. Along with ringing in the ears, one may also complain of headaches, irritability, restlessness, dizziness, red face, sore back, vomiting, or nausea.

Recommendations: black sesame seeds, black beans, walnuts, grapes, celery, oyster shells, pearl barley, azuki beans, Chinese black dates, yams, lotus seeds, chestnuts, chrysanthemum. Get plenty of sleep, massage the neck and head area, and try to live in a quiet, peaceful place, if possible.

Remedies:

1. Make tea from lotus seeds and chrysanthemums.

2. Make juice from celery and grapes, drink 1 c. 2 - 3 times daily.

3. Cook azuki beans and black beans with rice porridge and eat at least once daily.

4. Boil Chinese black dates, walnuts, and lotus seeds with rice porridge and eat once daily.

Avoid: loud noise, stress, tension, stimulating foods, spicy foods, smoking, alcohol, coffee

ULCERS (STOMACH OR DUODENUM)

Ulcers can occur anywhere along the food pathway, from the mouth to the stomach to the intestines. Ulcers can also occur in the vagina. The most common place for ulcers to occur are the stomach and duodenum (first part of the small intestines). Ulcers are characterized by burning pain. In the stomach, pain is usually worse on an empty stomach; if the ulcer is further down, there will be pain after meals. There may also be nausea. If the stools are black (digested blood), the ulcer is in the stomach or higher. If stools are red, the ulcer is lower than the stomach. If the red blood is mixed in the stool, the ulcer is in the small intestines. If red blood is on the stool then the ulcer is in the lower intestines or a result of a hemorrhoid.

Recommendations: potatoes, honey, cabbage, ginger, figs, papayas, squid bone, peanut oil, kale, persimmons

Remedies:

1. For mouth ulcers, apply the ash of charcoaled eggplant.

2. Drink potato juice daily on an empty stomach for at least 2 weeks.

3. Drink warm kale juice or cabbage juice on an empty stomach to help heal the ulcer.

4. Take 2 teaspoons peanut oil every morning on an empty stomach to help close the wound.

5. Drink fig juice.

6. Bake squid bone until crisp, powder it and take 1 teaspoon daily with honey.

7. Take blended papaya and milk or soy milk. Note, this remedy would not be good for a person with a lot of mucus,

dampness, or allergies, unless soy milk were substituted for the milk.

8. Take 2 tablespoons steamed honey on an empty stomach in the mornings.

9. Cook ginger (an amount the size of the thumb) with rice and have for breakfast every morning on an empty stomach.

10. Dry and charcoal persimmon and grind into powder; take 1 T. in a glass of warm water.

Avoid: spicy foods, hot foods, stimulants, shellfish, coffee, smoking, alcohol, fried foods, and stress

WORMS

This is a common condition among children. It can manifest in such symptoms as decreased appetite, abdominal pain, nausea, diarrhea or constipation, vomiting, anal itching at night and malnourished appearance. There are many types of worms including roundworms, pinworms, tapeworms, and hookworms.

Recommendations: pumpkin seeds, papaya seeds, coconut, garlic, hawthorn berries, sunflower seeds, Chinese prunes, ginger, vinegar, black pepper, walnut leaf

Remedies:
1. Make tea from 10 Chinese prunes, 6 g. black pepper and 3 slices fresh ginger. Drink 2 cups, an hour apart in the morning on an empty stomach. Do this every day for 1 week.

2. Take raw 1 T. pumpkin seeds, ground to powder, with warm water, twice in the morning an hour apart, every day for 1 week.

3. Eat 2 T. sunflower seeds every morning on an empty stomach.

4. Make tea from hawthorn berries and betel nuts and drink 2 cups in the morning on an empty stomach, 1 hour apart.

5. Charcoal black pepper, grind to powder, take 1/2 t. 3 times daily with warm water.

6. Make tea from betel nut and pumpkin seeds. Eat pumpkin seeds then drink the tea and within about 4 - 5 hours expect diarrhea and excretion of the worms.

7. Take the white part of green onion, make into juice and add 1 - 2 t. sesame oil; take 2 times daily on an empty stomach for 3 days.

8. Take coconut juice and 1/2 of a coconut every morning on an empty stomach; wait 3 hours before eating.

9. Take garlic on an empty stomach every morning.

10. Soak cotton with rice vinegar and plug up anus at night for three days, changing cotton each day. This will attract the worms to the anal area. Or do a rice vinegar enema and hold in all night; do this 3 days in a row.

11. Mash garlic and mix with vaseline, apply around anus every night for 3 days.

12. Mix raw garlic juice and rice vinegar with an equal part water and take on an empty stomach 3 days in a row.

13. Take 1 t. ground papaya seeds with warm water every morning on an empty stomach for 7 days.

Avoid: unsanitary foods, uncooked meats or fish, raw foods

SECTION

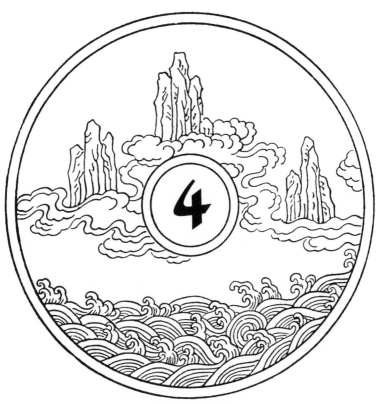

Simple Vegetarian Recipes

SIMPLE, VEGETARIAN RECIPES

These recipes are provided to serve as a guide to those wishing to move away from a heavily meat-based diet. Ideally, meat should comprise no more than 1/10 of the diet. Soy foods such as tofu, tempeh, soy milk and wheat gluten can provide good alternatives to animal products.

Cooking is an art. To do it well one must be creative, paying attention to how the combinations look as well as how they taste. Always choose foods according to what is seasonally available. Feel free to make substitutions in the recipes with this in mind. Let your taste buds guide you in the appropriate seasonings and combinations of dishes.

Some of the recipes call for *tamari*. This is a naturally aged soy sauce. *Miso* is a salty, aged soybean and grain paste, used for seasoning. Also used for seasoning is *Bragg's Liquid Aminos*; this is a low salt soy liquid, available in health food stores. *Kuzu* and *arrowroot* are thickening agents, similar to cornstarch. *Couscous* is a grain product that comes from the heart of duram wheat and is sweet in flavor.

Many of the recipes use sea vegetables such as *kombu, wakame, nori*, or *hiziki*. Sea vegetables (also known as seaweeds) should be included in the diet regularly for they are an excellent source of nutrients, particularly the minerals. They are also known to alkalinize the body, purify the blood, help dissolve fat and mucus deposits, and neutralize radioactive matter. Seaweeds come in a wide variety of shapes and sizes. The thin sheets called *nori* can be used to wrap grains or vegetables. *Wakame* and *kombu* are good soup additions. *Kombu* added to beans increases digestibility and decreases cooking time. One of the most flavorful sea vegetables is the red leafed *dulse*. The adventuresome may wish to try *arame* or *hiziki*; these look like thin black noodles, and are delicious with vegetables or tofu. *Agar flakes* can be used to make a gelatin-like dish called *kanten*.

In general, sea vegetables (except *nori*) need to be rinsed and soaked prior to using. For soups, just washing is sufficient. Dried seaweeds are always available in Oriental markets. Many delicious varieties from our northern Pacific waters are available in large health food stores.

In the recipes that follow, substitutions may be needed to follow a specific remedial diet. For example, a person with Candida yeast infection should leave out the tamari and miso (fermented foods) and substitute herb salt or some other seasoning. Someone with a *cold type* condition may need to add more warming foods to the recipes, such as scallions, garlic, ginger, or pepper. Those with *hot type* conditions may need to leave out the warming seasonings and so forth.

Imbalances can be well addressed by the addition of therapeutic herbs to the diet. Many of the herbs in the Chinese pharmacopeia were actually recognized as foods prior to their use as medicines. A few of the really delicious ones are lily bulbs, lycii berries, Chinese dioscorea yam, and jujube dates.The typical way of using these *food herbs* would be in soups, stews or grain dishes. The rich colors and textures add a great deal to the dish. For more information on cooking with Chinese herbs and specific recipes, we refer you to *101 Vegetarian Delights* by Lily Chuang and Cathy McNease and *Chinese Vegetarian Delights: Sugar and Dairy Free Cookbook* by Lily Chuang (both by SevenStar Communications)

The following common abbreviations are used:
t. is teaspoon
T. is tablespoon (3 teaspoons)
c. is cup (8 fluid ounces)

SOUPS
Sweet Squash and Seaweed Soup

1 stalk celery, diced
1 butternut squash (or other winter squash)
A few chopped leaves of Chinese cabbage
A small onion or bunch of scallions
1 small piece of wakame seaweed

Begin with 2 quarts water. Simmer the winter squash, peeled and diced, and the wakame, cut into small pieces. Add the onion and celery pieces. When the vegetables are tender, add 2 T. tamari or *Bragg's Liquid Aminos* and 3 T. garbanzo miso (or other light miso) which has been dissolved in a small amount of broth. Garnish with a sprig of cilantro. Serves 4.

Summer Vegetable Soup

1 onion
2 carrots
1 clove garlic
1 zucchini squash
2 tomatoes
1 handful green beans
1 cup fresh corn

Chop vegetables into small pieces; add to 2 quarts water. Cook until tender then add 1 c. tomato sauce, heat until warm. Season to taste with herb salt, tamari, or *Bragg's Liquid Aminos* and garnish with finely chopped cilantro and chives. Serves 4.

Soup Stock

4 6-8 inch pieces kombu seaweed
6 Chinese mushrooms

1 carrot
1 stalk celery
1 onion

Bring 2 quarts water to a boil with the above vegetables, then simmer for 1 hour. Strain and use the liquid for making soups or grains. It will store well in the refrigerator for about a week. Use the vegetables in some dish, perhaps a soup.

Black Bean Sauce or Soup

1 c. black beans
1 four inch piece kombu
1 small onion, finely chopped
2 garlic cloves
3 T. tamari
1 t. ginger juice
1/2 red bell pepper
2 T. cilantro

Soak beans overnight. Discard soak water, cover with fresh water and cook beans and kombu for about an hour. You may need to add more water.

During the last 20 minutes of cooking, add garlic, onions, and red bell pepper. Mix tamari and ginger juice in at the end. Blend for a creamy sauce to pour over grains or steamed vegetables. Serves 4.

Beet Sauce or Soup

5-6 carrots
2-3 large beets
2 onions
2-4 stalks celery
2 T. miso
3-4 cloves garlic

Cook vegetables with 3-4 cups water until tender. Blend vegetables with the cooking liquid. Add the miso, 2 T. olive oil, 1 t. basil and 1 t. oregano, and 1 t. umeboshi plum paste. Return to flame and simmer for 20 minutes to mix flavors. For sauce, add 2 T. arrowroot, cornstarch or kudzu, dissolved in 1/4 c. water to the mixture and heat until thick and smooth. Serve over noodles or steamed vegetables. Serves 4-6.

Chinese Noodle Soup

8 Chinese mushrooms, soaked with stems removed and sliced very thin
6 white mushrooms, sliced very thin
1 red bell pepper, sliced very thin
1 small yellow squash, sliced
1 small piece wakame, sliced into small pieces

Put vegetables into 2 quarts water or vegetable broth; cook until tender. Then add the following:
3 T. chopped cilantro
3 chopped green onions
1 T. tamari
1 t. peanut oil or toasted sesame oil
1 small handful bean threads (mung bean noodles)

Remove from fire and let sit, covered for 5 minutes. Serves 4.

Winter Melon Soup

3 qt. vegetable broth
3 c. chopped and peeled winter melon
2 carrots
2 celery stalks
1 onion
12 Chinese mushrooms, stems removed
6 oz. tofu noodles or finely sliced baked tofu

Cook together until tender, about 25 minutes. Then season with 1 t. chives, 1 T. tamari, and 1 t. peanut or sesame oil. Serves 4.

Creamy Split Pea Soup

1 c. green split peas
3 c. water
1 six inch piece kombu
1 carrot
1 celery stalk
1 small onion
1 t. tamari

Cook peas and kombu until soft. Add the vegetables and cook another 15 minutes. When vegetables are done, put in blender with the tamari, 1 T. cilantro, 1/4 t. paprika, 1/2 t. curry powder, 1/2 t. coriander seed powder, a pinch of nutmeg, and 1/2 c. almond or soy milk. Serves 4-6.

GRAIN DISHES
Fancy Rice

Cook brown rice as usual with 2 c. water to 1 c. dry rice. After about 25 minutes, add a finely chopped carrot, 3 chopped scallions, and 1/4 red bell pepper, finely chopped. Cook another 20 minutes or until water is all absorbed. Serves 2.

Nori Burritos

Toast sheets of nori seaweed briefly over the flame until it changes color from brown to green (this take about 15 seconds) or use *sushi nori* that has already been toasted. On one end, lay out cooked rice, chopped green onion, steamed carrot slices, pickled ginger, and crushed, toasted sesame seeds. Roll up like a burrito, moistening the edge to get it to stick. The edge can be moistened with tamari or *Bragg's Liquid Aminos* for added flavor.

Vegetable Pie

CRUST: Cook 1 c. brown rice with 2 3/4 c. water for 30 minutes, then add 1/2 c. couscous and cook another 10-15 minutes or until water is absorbed. When done, stir in the following:
1 c. grated jicama root
1 t. chives
1/2 t. basil
1/4 t. curry powder
1 t. tamari or *Bragg's Liquid Aminos*

Press into a pie pan and add the following, finely chopped:
6 oz. tempeh
2 small carrots
1 leek
1 celery stalk
5 Chinese mushrooms, soaked with stems removed

Steam the pie for 30 minutes. Garnish the top with chopped cilantro. Serves 4-6.

Millet Patties

Cook 1 c. millet in 3 c. water for 30 minutes, or until water is absorbed. Add 1/2 t. basil, 3 finely chopped scallions, 1 T. tamari, and 1/4 c. grated carrot; mix well. Put 2 inch wide patties on an oiled cookie sheet and bake at 325 degrees for 20-30 minutes. They should be crisp on the outside. Serves 4-6.

Stuffed Pumpkin

Cut the top off a small pumpkin; clean out the seeds and strings; save the lid. Fill with the following mixture:
3 c. cooked rice or barley
1 T. crushed, toasted sesame seeds
2-3 stalks celery, sliced
1 onion, finely chopped
1 T. parsley
1 t. thyme
1 t. sage
1/2 t. rosemary
1 T. tamari

Cover with lid and bake at 350 degrees for 1 1/4- 1 1/2 hours (until fork easily goes into pumpkin). Serves 4-6.

Simple Couscous Pie

1 c. couscous
1/4 c. amaranth or quinoa or millet (presoaked a few hours)
1 1/2 c. boiling water or broth
6 Chinese mushrooms, soaked and sliced
1 c. winter squash, mashed or grated
1 small leek
2 chard leaves
1/2 red bell pepper

Soak grains in the water 15 - 30 minutes, until soft. Mix with vegetables, all finely chopped. Press into a pie pan and top with chopped walnuts. Steam 40 minutes over medium flame. Serves 6.

Variations:
1. Substitute 1 c. fresh corn kernels for the yam.
2. Substitute 1 c. grated carrot for the squash.
3. Substitute 1 c. spinach for the chard.

This is an easily portable dish, good for lunch packs.

Basic Protein Cereal

1 c. brown rice (or 1/2 barley, 1/2 brown rice)
1/3 c. soy beans
1 T. sesame or sunflower seeds

Soak above in 3 c. water overnight or in hot water for a few hours. Pour into blender and blend well. Pour into a bowl and steam for 1 1/2 to 2 hours. Serves 4.

Variations:
1. Substitute black or azuki beans for the soy beans.
2. Substitute 1/2 c. millet for 1/2 c. rice.
3. Substitute walnuts or pecans for the sesames.
4. Season with ginger or cinnamon, or honey or rice syrup, or nut butter.
5. Substitute raw peanuts for the soy beans.

Chestnut Rice

1/2 c. dried chestnuts
1/3 c. raw peanuts
1 c. brown rice or sweet rice

Soak together the above with 3 3/4 c. water overnight or in hot water for several hours. Pour into a bowl and steam over low flame for 2 hours, stirring occasionally, until chestnuts are tender. Serves 4.

Variations:
1. Substitute walnuts for the chestnuts.
2. Substitute 1/2 c. barley for 1/2 c. rice.

Simple Grain Dish

1 c.whole grains (brown rice, barley, millet, sweet rice, couscous, or a mixture of these)
2 c. water

Mix grains and water and steam for 1 1/2 - 2 hours over a medium flame. Serves 2 - 4.

OR:

Use 1 c. grain to 2 - 2 1/2 c. water to cook grains directly over the flame (as opposed to steaming) for 45 - 50 minutes, or until the water is all absorbed.

Variations:

1. Add dates or raisins and cinnamon for seasoning.
2. Add steamed peanuts.
3. Add brown rice syrup or maple syrup.

The Fastest Cereal: Couscous

Pour 1 c. boiling water over 3/4 c. couscous. Let sit for 5 minutes, covered. Garnish with scallions and cilantro. Serves 2 - 4.

Variations:

1. Omit the scallions and cilantro and add a grated apple, 1/4 c. raisins, and a pinch of cinnamon.
2. Add steamed peanuts.
3. Add 1/2 c. grated carrots, and a pinch of ginger.

Steamed Corn Bread

1 c. grated apple (or chopped fresh pineapple)
2 c. coconut milk or soy milk or almond milk or pineapple-coconut juice
1 medium banana
1/3 c. whole wheat flour
1 c. cornmeal
1/2 c. oatmeal or millet flour or brown rice flour
1/8 c. lycii berries or raisins (optional)

Blend the liquid with the banana. Add the rest of the ingredients and mix well. Pour into a pie plate and steam 30 minutes over medium flame. It is done when a chopstick inserted in the center comes out clean. Serves 6.

Variations:

1. Substitute 1 c. grated carrot for the apple or use 1/2 carrot and 1/2 apple.
2. Add a pinch of each cinnamon, ginger, and nutmeg.
3. Add 1/4 c. coconut.

The following recipe is reprinted courtesy of Lily Chuang from her cookbook, *Chinese Vegetarian Delights: Sugar and Dairy Free Cookbook* (SevenStar Communications):

Mochi

Soak 2 c. brown or black sweet rice in 2 c. water. Then put in blender, a little bit at a time. Continue until all is blended.

OR: Combine 2 c. powdered brown or black sweet rice and 2 c. water. Mix together well.

Steam for 1 1/2 hours on medium flame, covered. Open and stir well about 1/2 hour before it is done. Let the rice paste cool.

Use wet hands to handle the rice paste. Form a small ball, flatten between hands, and put a small amount of one of the following fillings in the center: a combination of chopped, cooked Chinese mushrooms, seaweed, baked tofu, and seasoning; bean paste (azuki, black, or mung - good in summer); nut butter; or raisins. For a sweeter variety, fill with bean paste and honey or rice syrup; this makes an excellent dessert.

Close the patty and form a ball. Roll in one of the following: sunflower, sesame, or cashew meal, coconut, carob powder, or toasted soybean flour. Serves 4 - 6.

The following recipe is reprinted courtesy of Lily Chuang and Cathy McNease from *101 Vegetarian Delights* (SevenStar Communications):

Sweet Breakfast Porridge

3/4 c. brown rice
1/4 c. barley flakes
1/2 c. raw skinless peanuts
10 Chinese jujube dates
1 slice fresh ginger root

Cook all ingredients with 5 c. of water in a crockpot overnight, or on the stove for 2 1/2 - 3 hours on low; stir occasionally. Serves 4.

BEAN AND TOFU DISHES
Tofu and Mushroom Casserole

2 lb. plain tofu, lightly steamed
12 large Chinese mushrooms, soaked until soft, thin sliced
2 c. pea pods
1 bunch scallions

Slice tofu into 1/2 inch slices and put in bottom of rectangular baking dish. Lightly simmer mushrooms then add pea pods and scallions for last 5 minutes. Put these vegetables on top of the tofu. Use the vegetable cooking water plus enough water to make 3 c. liquid. Add 2 T. tamari or *Bragg's Liquid Aminos*. Dissolve 3 T. kudzu, arrowroot, or cornstarch in a small amount of liquid; add to the rest of the liquid and simmer, stirring often until the liquid thickens. Pour this gravy on top of the tofu and vegetable mixture. Garnish with crushed, toasted almonds and finely chopped cilantro. Serves 4.

Azuki Bean and Squash Casserole

1 c. azuki beans, soaked overnight
2 6-8 inch pieces of kombu
1 small butternut squash or other winter squash

Cover beans and kombu with water and simmer about 1 hour, adding water if needed. Then add the cubed and peeled squash. Cook until tender, about 1/2 hour. Stir in a pinch of sea salt or 1-2 teaspoons tamari. Serves 4.

Clinton's Savory Azuki Beans with Chestnuts

1 c. azuki beans, soaked overnight
1/4 c. dried chestnuts, soaked 1 hour
1 six inch strip kombu seaweed
1 t. lycii berries (optional)

Soak azuki beans overnight; discard soak water. Place kombu in pot then add chestnuts and beans. Cover with 2 inches water and bring to a boil. Simmer 2-3 hours, adding enough water to keep beans covered. Add a pinch of sea salt or 1 t. tamari and the lycii berries 10-15 minutes before done cooking. Serves 4.

Tofu Skins and Mushrooms

Soak 12 strips of dried tofu skin (available in Oriental grocery stores) and 6 Chinese mushrooms in 4-6 cups water plus 2 T. tamari for at least 4 hours. Then tie each strip in a knot, and simmer with the mushrooms, thinly sliced, for 20 minutes. Add 8 sliced, white mushrooms and a sliced red bell pepper and continue to simmer another 10-15 minutes.

Pour off the liquid and thicken it with 1-2 T. kudzu or arrowroot (do this in a separate pan, heating until thick). Pour the sauce over the tofu and mushroom mixture and serve over steamed greens. Serves 4.

Steamed Peanuts

Soak 1 c. raw peanuts in 2 c. water overnight or in hot water for a few hours. Steam with soak water for 1 1/2 - 2 hours over medium flame. This makes a delicious, nutritious addition to cereals, vegetable dishes, and grains.

Scrambled Tofu

1/2 lb. tofu
2 stalks celery
6 white mushrooms
1 tomato

Chop vegetables finely. Saute in 1/4 c. water or 1 T. oil. When almost done, add crumbled tofu. Let heat for 5 - 10 minutes. Season with 1 t. tamari soy sauce.

Variations:
1. Substitute 1 beaten egg for 1/2 of the tofu.
2. Substitute 1 small zucchini squash for the mushrooms.

Tofu with Seaweed

1 package baked tofu, sliced or 1/2 lb. plain tofu, cubed
1 handful hiziki or arame seaweed, soaked in hot water 20 - 30 minutes
1 large carrot, diced
1/2 c. jicama, diced
1 small onion, chopped
4 Chinese mushrooms, presoaked and sliced

Stir fry carrots, onions, mushrooms then jicama in small amount of water (or mushrooms soak water). When almost done, add the tofu and seaweed. Cover and let steam for 5 - 10 minutes. Season to taste with tamari soy sauce and toasted sesame oil.

Variation:
1. Substitute wakame or kombu for the hiziki. Note these need to be presoaked for 1-2 hours.
2. Add diced burdock root (gobo) at the beginning with the carrots.
3. Use white mushrooms instead of the Chinese ones.

Tofu Dressing

1/2 lb. plain tofu
1/4 c. oil
1 T. lemon juice
1 t. honey or rice syrup
1 t. rice or apple cider vinegar 1/2 t. tamari soy sauce (or a pinch of salt)1 T. sesame tahini

Blend until creamy. Use on salads, vegetables, or sandwiches.

Variations:
1. Add 1/4 c. poppy seeds.
2. Add 1 1/2 t. prepared mustard.
3. Add 1/2 t. basil and 1/4 t. garlic powder.
4. Add 2 whole green onions.

MISCELLANEOUS RECIPES
Sesame Seed Garnish

Wash 2 c. whole, brown sesame seeds. Toast in dry skillet, stirring often until seeds can be easily crushed between the fingers. Separately, heat 1/2 t. sea salt in dry skillet until the chlorine gas is removed (you will smell it). Then mix sesame seeds and salt and grind in blender or in mortar and pestle. Store in the refrigerator. Use as a garnish for a strong nutty flavor. The salt can be omitted if desired; kelp powder may be substituted for the salt.

Basic Vegetable Stir Fry

Use a variety of vegetables, diced or sliced. Stir fry in a small amount of water or broth, covered, the slower cooking vegetables first (i.e. carrots, green beans, cauliflower, etc.), then add the faster cooking ones (i.e. jicama, zucchini squash, broccoli, etc.) When the last vegetables go in, you can add tofu or gluten pieces also. Presoaked seaweeds can be added near the beginning.

When everything is done, season to taste with oil, soy sauce (or *Bragg's Liquid Aminos* or herb salt) or your favorite cooking herbs. Basil and cilantro are particularly good with vegetables.

Variations:
1. Add steamed peanuts or almonds.
2. Add 1 clove of garlic at the beginning.
3. Add finely grated ginger toward the end of the cooking.
4. Add chopped green onions at the end.
5. Add Chinese mushrooms (presoaked) at the beginning.

Almond Stir Fry

1 small yam
1 small head cauliflower
1 leek or onion
2 summer squash
1 handful green beans
1/4 lb. white mushrooms

Chop vegetables into small pieces. Put in skillet with about 1/4 inch water. Cover and steam until vegetables are tender. Pour out any remaining water into a bowl. Add 1 T. arrowroot or cornstarch and stir until dissolved; pour back into vegetables and heat briefly until liquid thickens. Stir in 1/2-3/4 c. crushed, roasted almonds and 1/2 t. toasted sesame oil. Serves 2-4.

Stir Fry Over Noodles

2 c. chopped broccoli
1 red bell pepper
2 garlic cloves
1 zucchini
2 leeks
1 carrot
5 white mushrooms

Heat 1 T. peanut oil; saute the garlic and leeks. Then add mushrooms, carrots, broccoli, and 1/4 c. water or broth. Cover and cook 5 minutes. Last add zucchini and red bell pepper and cook another 5 minutes. Season to taste with basil, cilantro, and tamari. Serve over whole wheat or rice noodles. Serves 2-4.

Almond Milk

Soak 1 c. raw almonds for at least 4 hours. Grind in blender with 2 c. water, strain and put the solids back in the blender and repeat the process 2 more times. Combining all of the strained *milk* there should be a total of 6 c. Put some of the liquid back in the blender with 1/2 t. vanilla or almond extract, a pinch of cinnamon, and 2 T. honey or maple syrup. Blend and mix back into the other liquid. Store in the refrigerator and use within a few days. Almond milk can also be sweetened by grinding in 5-6 dates or a small handful of raisins. This same procedure can be used to make other *nut milks* like cashew or sesame *milk*.

Soy bean Milk

Soak 1 c. soy beans at least 8 hours, or as long as 3 days in the refrigerator. Blend soaked beans with 3 c. water, then strain through a cloth, squeezing out the milk. Put the pulp back in the blender with more water and repeat the process until you have 1 1/2 quarts of *soy milk*. Bring to a boil and simmer for 15-20 minutes, stirring often to prevent sticking and boiling over. Soy milk can be used plain, mixed with carob powder and rice syrup, or blended with fruits such as papaya or banana (cool soy milk before mixing with fruit).

Protein Pudding

3 c. soy milk
1/3 c. rice syrup (or maple syrup)
1 bar agar seaweed

Rinse agar then mix with soy milk. Cook together until agar is dissolved. Mix in syrup. Pour into dishes and let firm.

Variations:
1. Add 1/2 c. raisins or chopped dates.
2. Add 1/2 c. pecans, sunflower seeds, walnuts, or cashews.
3. Flavor with 1/2 t. vanilla or 3 T. carob powder.
4. Substitute almond milk for the soy milk and garnish the top with 1/4 c. almonds when almost firm.

Pecan Pudding

2 c. soy bean milk
1/2 c. pecans or walnuts
1/4 - 1/3 c. maple or brown rice syrup
3 T. arrowroot or kudzu or sweet rice flour
2 T. carob powder

Blend all ingredients well. Then heat over low flame until thickened, stirring constantly. Serve warm.

Wheat Gluten (Wheat Meat)

2 1/2 pounds gluten flour (or unbleached white flour or whole wheat flour)
1 quart water

Mix together to form a stiff dough. Then cover and let sit for one hour. Then put the bowl in the sink with the faucet on low and wash out the starch. Continue kneading the dough and pouring off the starchy white water until the water is clear. This will take many washings and much kneading (about 10 minutes).

While washing the gluten, simmer the following broth: 2 quarts water, 3 small strips kombu seaweed, 1/3 c. tamari, 4 Chinese mushrooms and several slices of fresh ginger (onion, garlic, or bay leaf can also be used). When the broth has simmered 30 minutes, spoon out the solids.

With the broth at a mild boil, drop in small (1") gluten pieces. When they rise to the top they are done. The longer gluten cooks, the more tender it will become. For stronger flavored gluten, it can be marinated (soaked) in the seasoning broth for several hours after cooking. Gluten freezes well if you make a large batch. Gluten can be used whenever a *meaty* textured protein food is desired.

Basic Tomato Sauce

3 c. chopped tomatoes
1 bell pepper
1 garlic clove
1 small onion

Cook the above until tender. Then put in blender with 2 T. fresh basil or 1/2 T. dried basil, and 1/2 t. oregano, 1 t.

onion powder, and 1 1/2 T. tamari. Return to pan when well blended.

Stir 2 T. arrowroot or cornstarch or kudzu into a small amount of water. Add to the tomato mixture, and heat, stirring often, until thick.

Variations:
1. Add 1/2 c. sauteed white mushrooms.
2. Add 1/2 c. zucchini.
3. Serve over noodles or steamed spaghetti squash.

Simple Oil and Vinegar Dressing

Blend 1/2 c. each of oil and vinegar (rice or apple cider) or lemon juice and 1 T. tamari or *Bragg's Liquid Aminos*. You can also blend in 1/4 t. garlic or onion powder. To make **Italian Dressing,** add 1/2 t. oregano and 1/2 t. basil.

Sprouts

Sprouts are easy to grow and very nutritious. The nutritional value of sprouts is increased manyfold over the unsprouted seeds.

RAINBOW MIX: This is a blend of azuki beans, mung beans, and lentils. Soak seeds (together or separately) overnight. Pour off the soak water and rinse 2 times daily. A jar with a screen on top is very handy for growing sprouts. Store in a warm, dark place 3 - 5 days (remembering to rinse twice daily). At the end of growth period, put in sunlight for 30 - 60 minutes, for the leaves to produce chlorophyll. These can be used raw or lightly sauteed. Whole peas or whole wheat may also be added to this mix.

LIGHT MIX: This blend is alfalfa seeds, red clover seeds, and daikon radish seeds (optional). Sprout these in the same fashion as above. These sprouts are used raw as a garnish for salads and sandwiches.

Sandwich Fillings

These fillings can be used with any whole grain bread or pita (pocket) breads or rolled inside of whole wheat tortillas (chapatis).

1. RAINBOW SPROUTS: Saute lightly in water or oil, mung, azuki and lentil sprouts, grated carrot, shredded red cabbage, soaked hiziki seaweed, and grated ginger.

2. GARBANZO SPREAD: Cook garbanzo beans until soft then mash and mix with sesame tahini, lemon juice, garlic powder, and a pinch of salt. Garnish with alfalfa/clover sprouts and tomato slices.

3. NUT BUTTER: Almond butter, sesame butter, or cashew butter, grated carrots, green onions, and cilantro.

4. SOY BURGER: Combine cooked soy and garbanzo beans, grated carrots, sliced mushrooms and enough cornstarch or arrowroot or flour to hold together. Steam for 15 - 20 minutes over medium flame.

5. SWEET TREAT: Combine almond butter, rice syrup, grated apple, and a pinch of ginger or cinnamon.

6. EGGPLANT SPREAD: Steam eggplant until soft. Mash and mix with sesame tahini, garlic, and lemon juice.

7. COLORFUL SANDWICH: Steam beets and carrots. Mash and mix with sauteed, finely chopped, tofu cabbage, and celery.

SECTION

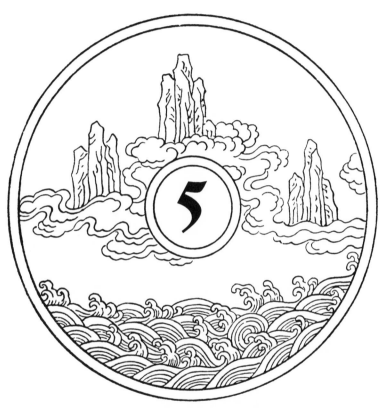

Sample
Meal Plan

SAMPLE MEAL PLAN

Our meal plan is intended to provide some direction in nutritional meal planning. It is not meant to be a rigid regimen, rather a framework within which to plan your meals. Feel free to make substitutions to suit your needs. If your diet includes fish and meat, substitute for the tofu or other soy products up to 10% of the diet. If your diet includes eggs or dairy products, those too could be substituted as protein sources.

In general, each meal will be constructed around a grain food with fresh vegetables and fruits. As a vegetarian it is important to eat a variety of bean foods also to provide a more balanced protein than grain alone. Examples are soy bean milk over oatmeal, lentils and rice, or black bean soup with corn bread. Dairy products, eggs, nuts and seeds are also used to complement grain or bean protein.

Breakfast should sustain us through the first portion of our productive day, so don't skimp there. Lunch is usually lighter because of the typical time frame within which we have to eat midday, although this is an ideal time for the biggest meal of the day. Dinner time is usually more leisurely, and allows for more creativity in the kitchen. Try not to overeat before bedtime.

For the Spring/Summer meals we will tend to eat lighter and include more fresh fruits and cooling foods. Moister foods will be needed during hot and dry seasons. Fall/Winter meals need to provide extra fuel to sustain our energy and keep us warm. We will tend toward more baked and warming foods during the cold seasons.

SPRING/SUMMER MEALS

BREAKFAST	LUNCH	DINNER
Monday		
Cream of rice or wheat with raisins and cinnamon	Winter melon soup with tofu*	Stir fried vegetables with tofu and gluten*
Steamed apple	Rice cake with nut butter	Brown rice*
Tuesday		
Scrambled tofu with tomato and zucchini*	Chinese noodle soup*	Baked yam
Brown rice with pecans	Couscous with steamed peanuts*	Tofu with seaweed*
	Papaya slices	Fancy rice*
Wednesday		
Apple/banana/carrot corn bread*	Fruit salad with soy yogurt and almonds	Tomato-mushroom sauce over whole wheat noodles and tempeh cubes*
Soy milk*	Brown rice drink (amasake)	Steamed broccoli
Thursday		
Couscous with grated apples and raisins*	Nori rolls with rice, steamed carrots and cilantro*	Vegetable tofu stir fry*
Almond milk*		Mochi rice balls*

Friday

Steamed pineapple
corn bread*

Almond Pudding*

Pita bread with
rainbow sprouts
and carrots*

Green salad/
tofu dressing*

Tofu skins and
mushrooms*

Brown rice*

Steamed eggplant

Saturday

Simple cereal with
dates, raisins,
and sunflower
seeds*

Summer vegetable
soup*

Chapatis with
avocado, sprouts

Couscous-corn
pie*

Green salad with
sesame garnish*

Sunday

Scrambled tofu
with egg*

Couscous pie*

Soy Milk*

Garbonzo spread
on whole wheat
bread*

Apple slices

Vegetable stir
fry*

Protein cereal
with peanuts and
pecans*

Those foods that are marked by an asterisk (*) are listed in the recipe section with detailed instructions on preparation.

FALL/WINTER MEALS

Breakfast	Lunch	Dinner
Monday		
Basic protein cereal with azuki or black beans	Stir fry vegetables with tofu and seaweed*	Tofu skins with Chinese mushrooms*
Steamed tofu with ginger, soy sauce, and nut meal	Simple grain dish*	Rice/barley/couscous*
		Steamed broccoli
Tuesday		
Simple cereal with dates, raisins, and peanuts*	Soyburger sandwich*	Couscous-corn pie*
Steamed corn bread with sesame butter and rice syrup*	Vegetable soup*	Azuki beans and chestnuts*
		Steamed spinach
Wednesday		
Simple cereal with ginger, scallions, and miso*	Nori burritos* casserole*	Tofu-mushroom
Steamed broccoli and green beans	Black bean soup*	Stuffed pumpkin*
		Pecan pudding*
Soy milk*		

Thursday

Steamed corn bread
with black bean
spread and sliced
banana*

Soy milk with carob*

Vegetable pie*

Steamed greens

Cashew stir fry*

Millet and rice*

Protein pudding*

Friday

Steamed corn,
beets, and spinach

Pita bread sand-
wiches with mochi*

Cinnamon soy milk*

Stir fry vege-
tables over
noodles*

Sweet squash and
seaweed soup*

Azuki bean and
squash casserole*

Sweet brown rice
and couscous*

Cauliflower

Saturday

Simple cereal with
tempeh, mushrooms,
and celery*

Steamed apples

Creamy split pea
soup*

Millet patties*

Beet sauce over
noodles*

Tofu and Chinese
mushrooms*

Sunday

Chestnut rice with
peanuts*

Steamed carrots

Soy milk*

Chapatis with
rainbow sprouts
and carrots*

Steamed yam

Black bean
over rice*

Vegetable stir
fry*

SECTION

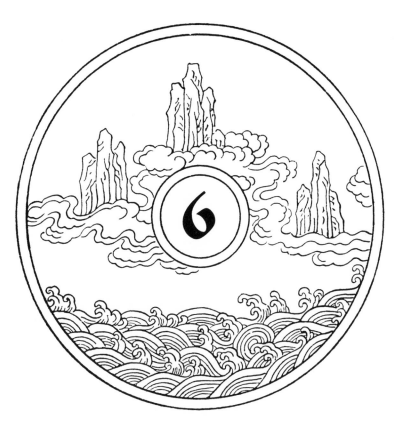

Appendices

GLOSSARY

Astringent - substance that has a constricting action or causes contraction of orifices. Examples of astringent action are to stop sweating or stop diarrhea.

Arteriosclerosis - hardening of the arteries, usually due to aging or high consumption of fatty foods over a long period of time.

Ascites - accumulation of fluids in the abdomen, usually due to cirrhosis of the liver.

Carminative - substance that promotes normal flow of energy and removes obstructions; substance that relieves gas from the gastrointestinal tract.

Chi (Qi) - energy or life force; an entity that denotes the functional aspect of the body in Chinese Medicine.

Chi (Qi) Gong - a set of breathing exercises for strengthening and balancing the energy (Chi), relaxing the mind, and for the purpose of maintaining health and curing disease.

Clears heat - to remove or neutralize pathogenic heat from the body; to soothe a hot, feverish condition with cooling foods or herbs.

Colitis - inflammation of the colon.

Cold-type condition - a condition caused by cold, one of the six pathogenic factors in the environment, or simply the result of not enough fire (Yang) in the body. It is benefitted by application of warmth (i.e. heating pad) or warming foods and herbs and aggravated by cold.

Cold-type person - one who tends to feel cold a lot, be pale-complexioned, lack energy, tend toward loose stools. (For a more thorough list of symptoms, refer to page 7 of text.)

Conjunctivitis - inflammation and infection of the mucous membranes of the eyelids as a result of too much heat in the body, specifically in the Liver, according to Chinese Medicine.

Consolidate (the lungs) - to strengthen the lungs in conditions of chronic cough, asthma and shortness of breath.

Cooling food - a food that has a counteracting effect to heat in the body, i.e., elicits a cooling response from the body; food of a Yin nature; food that lowers metabolism.

Dampness - one of the external causes of disease that disturbs the normal flow of energy and particularly the digestive functioning of the Spleen and Stomach, characterized by heaviness, stagnation, and turbidity; fluid accumulation due to impaired water metabolism.

Deficiency - condition of weakness or lack of either energy or substance due to illness or improper lifestyle, diet, or mental attitude.

Descend - to move energy in a downward direction in the body.

Disharmony - imbalance or disease or lack of healthy function.

Diuresis - a process that promotes smooth urination and reduces edema.

Diuretic - a food or herb that promotes urination in order to relieve swelling or discomfort in urination.

Diaphoretic- a substance that induces perspiration in order to expel pathogenic factors and toxins.

Dryness - one of the six pathogenic factors in the environment. Disorders with dryness are associated with thirst, dry mouth and throat, fever, constipation, scanty concentrated urine, dry cough, and emaciation. This can also be due to internal imbalance in the body.

Dysentery - Extreme diarrhea and tenesmus due to bacterial or viral infection.

Dysuria - painful or difficult urination.

Edema - abnormal accumulation of fluids in the body; swelling.

Essence ("Jing") - the source of life, found in eggs, sperms, marrow, and the brain and stored in the Kidneys; provides for growth, development and reproduction throughout one's entire lifetime.

Five Element Theory - an ancient philosophical concept to explain the phenomena of energy transformation and the composition and relationships of the natural world and the human body. A further refinement of the concept of opposites (Yin and Yang) into four degrees, the fifth being the center or balance. (For a more thorough understanding of the five element theory, please refer to *Tao, The Subtle Universal Law* by Ni, Hua-Ching.)

Gastritis - inflammation of the stomach.

Gruel (congee or porridge) - grain that has been cooked with extra water and cooking time to the point of being *soupy.*

Harmonize - restore general balance; to bring together into smooth functioning.

Hot-type condition - condition that is usually caused by heat, one of the six pathogenic factors in the environment, or a lack of water (Yin) to counterbalance the fire (Yang) in the body. It is benefitted by cooling foods and treatment, and aggravated by heat. This is usually an acute, excess condition, i.e., infections, fevers, and boils.

Hot-type person - one who tends to feel hot a lot, sweat freely, be red in face or tongue, have an excess of energy, be thirsty. (For a more complete list of symptoms, refer to page 7 in the text.)

Hypertension - high blood pressure.

Lactostasis - hampered milk production or secretion due to physical or functional obstruction.

Leukorrhea - white or yellow mucous discharge from the cervix or the vagina.

Liver heat (or fire) rising - a condition in which an excessive amount of heat in the Liver rises to the upper part of the body causing red painful eyes, flushed cheeks, headache, fits of anger, emotional instability, dizziness, ringing in the ears, and insomnia.

Neurasthenia - nervous exhaustion characterized by fatigue, weakness, headache, sweating, polyuria, tinnitus, dizziness, fear, photophobia, and insomnia.

Pathogen - a microorganism or substance capable of producing a disease. In Chinese Medicine it refers to anything that may cause imbalance within the body including environmental factors (wind, cold, heat, dampness, dryness, summer heat) and emotions.

Rebellious Chi - energy that moves upwardly when it normally should be going down, i.e., coughing, vomiting, and hiccupping.

Shen - spirit.

Stagnancy - a sluggishness or impeded circulation of blood, Chi, or body fluids.

Summer heat - one of the external causes of disease characterized by irritability, fever, headache, thirst, restlessness, and sweating.

T'ai Chi Ch'uan - an ancient Chinese exercise for harmonizing the mind, body, and spirit, whose connected movements somewhat resemble a graceful dance.

Tonify - to strengthen or build.

Toxins - poisons; in Chinese Medicine this term often refers to the presence of bacteria or virus.

Ventilate (lungs) - to disperse energy stagnation in the lungs and to soothe breathing and help relieve cough and asthma.

Visceras - internal organs.

Warming food - one that reduce coldness in the body or is of a Yang nature; food that raises metabolism.

Wind - one of the external causes of diseases; a syndrome characterized by fever, chills, head and body ache. Internal wind can disrupt the balance and manifest such symptoms as dizziness, fainting, convulsions, tremor, numbness, or pain that moves around (like the wind).

Wind-cold - common cold or flu caused by the invasion of wind and cold. Symptoms are severe chills, mild fever, head and body ache, no sweat, and sinus congestion.

Wind-heat - common cold or flu caused by the invasion of wind and heat. Symptoms are high fever, mild chills, sore throat, body and headache sweating, thirst.

Yang - relating to the male, active, positive, fiery, energetic side of life or nature of a person.

Yang deficiency - a lack of heat or fire (Yang) within the body to counterbalance the water (Yin), characterized by coldness, Chi deficiency, tiredness, diarrhea with watery stools; a lack of energy to balance bodily substance.

Yin - relating to the female, passive, negative, watery, cool, substance side of life or nature of a person.

Yin deficiency - a lack of the coolness or water (Yin) within the body to counterbalance the fire (Yang), usually resulting in heat symptoms such as irritability, red cheeks, night sweats, dry cough, dry throat and insomnia; a lack of bodily substance to balance energy

CHART 1: ENERGETIC PROPERTIES OF FOODS

C O L D   C O O L

V E G E T A B L E S

COLD	COOL	
Chinese cabbage	alfalfa sprout	dandelion greens
mung bean sprout	asparagus	eggplant
seaweed	bamboo shoot	endive lettuce
snow pea	beet	lotus root
water chestnut	bok choy	potato
white mushroom	broccoli	pumpkin
	burdock root	romaine lettuce
	button mushroom	soy bean sprout
	cabbage	spinach
	carrot	summer squash
	cauliflower	turnip
	celery	winter melon
	corn	watercress
	cucumber	winter squash
	daikon radish	zucchini

F R U I T S

COLD	COOL
banana	apple
cantaloupe	apricot
grapefruit	fig
mulberry	lemon
pear	orange
pear-apple	peach
watermelon	persimmon
	strawberry
	tomato

G R A I N S

millet
pearl barley
white rice
wheat

NEUTRAL   WARM   H O T

V E G E T A B L E S

NEUTRAL	WARM	HOT
chard	bell pepper	garlic
lettuce	Chinese chive	scallion
Shitake mushroom	Ganoderma mush-room	
sweet potato		
taro root	green bean	
yam	kale	
	leek	
	mustard green	
	onion	
	parsley	
	parsnip	

F R U I T S

NEUTRAL	WARM
Chinese date	cherry
loquat	Chinese prune
mango	coconut
olive	dried papaya
papaya	grape
	hawthorn berry
	litchi (lychee)
	pineapple
	plum
	raspberry
	tangerine

G R A I N S

NEUTRAL	WARM
buckwheat	oats
brown rice	sweet rice
corn meal	wheat bran
rice bran	wheat germ
rye	

C O L D C O O L

S E E D S A N D B E A N S

pumpkin seed

mung bean
soy bean
tofu
winter melon seed

A N I M A L P R O D U C T S

pork

chicken egg
clam
crab

H E R B S

bamboo shavings
cassia seeds
Chinese cucumber
chrysanthemum
goldenseal root
honeysuckle flower
lily bulb
motherwort leaf
mulberry leaf
oyster shell
reed root

American ginseng
cilantro
corn silk
kudzu (pueraria)
mint leaf
pueraria root

M I S C E L L A N E O U S

salt
vitamin C
white sugar

tea

NEUTRAL   WARM   HOT

S E E D S   A N D   B E A N S

NEUTRAL	WARM
almond	black bean
azuki bean	brown sesame seed
black sesame seed	chestnut
filbert	lentil
kidney bean	pine nut
lotus seed	walnut
peanut	
pea	
sunflower seed	

A N I M A L   P R O D U C T S

NEUTRAL	WARM	HOT
fish (ocean)	beef	lamb
gelatin	chicken	
dairy products	fish (freshwater)	
oyster	shrimp	
	turkey	

H E R B S

NEUTRAL	WARM	HOT
Chinese yam	anise seed	black pepper
licorice root	basil	cinnamon bark
lycii berry	cardamon seed	dry ginger
poria mushroom	carob pod	
	citrus peels	
	clove	
	coriander seed	
	Dang Gui	
	fennel seed	
	fresh ginger	
	Oriental ginseng	

M I S C E L L A N E O U S

NEUTRAL	WARM
barley malt	brown sugar
rice malt	coffee
black fungus	molasses
honey	rice vinegar
white fungus	wine

CHART 2: 5 ELEMENTS CORRESPONDENCES

	WOOD	FIRE
ORGANS:	LIVER, GALL BLADDER	HEART, SMALL INTESTINE PERICARDIUM, SANJIAO
FLAVOR:	SOUR	BITTER
SENSE:	SIGHT-EYES	TASTE-TONGUE
COLOR:	GREEN	RED
EMOTION:	ANGER	JOY (MANIA)
VOICE:	SHOUTING	LAUGHTER
PHYSICAL MANIFESTATION:	MUSCLES AND TENDONS	BLOOD VESSELS
MODE OF ACTION:	TWITCHING	ITCHING
INTERNAL ENERGY:	HUN CHI (PSYCHIC ENERGY)	SHEN CHI (DIRECTING CHI)
BODY FLUID:	BILE AND TEARS	BLOOD AND SWEAT
CLIMATE:	WIND	HEAT
SEASON:	SPRING	SUMMER
ORIENTATION:	EAST	SOUTH
DEVELOPMENT:	BIRTH	GROWTH
NEGATIVE DRIVE:	HOSTILITY	GREED
CORRUPTING INFLUENCE:	COMPETITION	SEX
ATTRIBUTES OF MIND:	RATIONALITY	SPIRITUALITY
MORAL:	BENEVOLENCE	HUMILITY

EARTH	METAL	WATER
SPLEEN, STOMACH, PANCREAS	LUNGS, LARGE INTESTINES	KIDNEYS, BLADDER
SWEET	PUNGENT	SALTY
TOUCH - SKIN	SMELL - NOSE	HEARING - EARS
YELLOW	WHITE	BLACK
WORRY	SADNESS	FEAR
SINGING	CRYING	GROANING
FLESH	SKIN AND BODY HAIR	BONE
HICCUPPING	COUGHING	SHIVERING
YUAN CHI (PRIMAL CHI)	PO CHI (PHYSICAL CHI)	CHING CHI (CREATIVE QI)
SALIVA	JIN (MUCOUS SECRETIONS)	SEXUAL FLUIDS
HUMIDITY	DRYNESS	COLD
LATE SUMMER (AND PERIOD BETWEEN SEASONS)	AUTUMN	WINTER
CENTER	WEST	NORTH
MATURITY	HARVEST	STORAGE
AMBITION	STUBBORNNESS	DESIRE
MIND	MONEY	ALCOHOL
TRANQUILITY	SENTIMENTALITY	DESIRE
TRUSTFULNESS	RECTITUDE	WISDOM

CHART 3: 5 ENERGETIC TRANSFORMATIONS

THE CREATION CYCLE

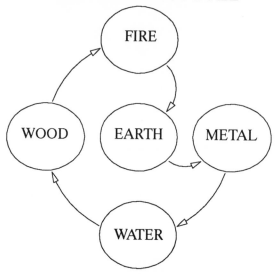

THE CONTROL CYCLE

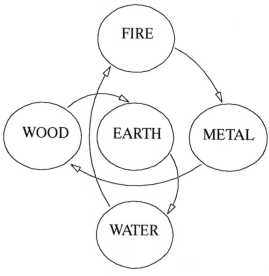

BIBLIOGRAPHY

For further reading on the subjects of Traditional Chinese Medicine, Chinese Nutrition, and the Taoist healing arts, we suggest the following books. Those books marked by an asterisk (*) are suggested for further information on Chinese Herbs.

*Beinfield, Harriet and Efrem Korngold. *Between Heaven and Earth: A Guide to Chinese Medicine.* New York: Ballantine Books, 1991.

*Bensky, Dan and Randall Barolet. *Chinese Herbal Medicine: Formulas and Strategies.* Seattle, Washington: Eastland Press, 1990.

*Bensky, Dan and Andrew Gamble. *Chinese Herbal Medicine: Materia Medica.* Seattle, Washington: Eastland Press, 1986.

Butt, Gary and Freena Bloomfield. *Harmony Rules.* London: Arrow Books, Ltd., 1985.

Colbin, Annemarie. *Food and Healing.* New York: Ballantine Books, 1986.

Essentials of Chinese Acupuncture. Beijing, China: Foreign Language Press, 1980.

Flaws, Bob and Honora Wolfe. *Prince Wen Hui's Cook: Chinese Dietary Therapy.* Brookline, Massachusetts: Paradigm Publications, 1983.

*Gallagher, Paul. *Chinese Herbal and Dietary Therapy.* *Yoga Journal*, Issue 67 (March-April, 1986), 33-36.

Haas, Elson. *Staying Healthy With the Seasons.* Berkeley, California: Celestial Arts, 1981.

Jou, Tsung Hwa. *The Tao of T'ai Chi Ch'uan: Way to Rejuvenation.* Piscataway, New Jersey: T'ai Chi Foundation, 1983.

220

Kaptchuk, Ted J. *The Web That Has No Weaver.* New York: Congdon and Weed, 1983.

*Leung, Albert Y. *Chinese Herbal Remedies.* New York: Universe Books, 1984.

Liu, Da. *Taoist Health Exercises Book.* New York: Perigee Books, 1983.

Lu, Henry C. *Chinese System of Food Cures.* New York: Sterling Publishing Co., 1986.

Maciocia, Giovanni. *The Foundations of Chinese Medicine.* New York: Churchill Livingstone, 1989.

*Ming-Dao, Deng. *Scholar Warrior: An Introduction* to *the Tao in Everyday Life.* San Francisco: Harpercollins, 1990.

Ni, Hua Ching. *8000 Years of Wisdom: Conversations With Taoist Master Ni, Hua Ching, Vol. 1.* Santa Monica, California: SevenStar Communications, 1983.

Ni, Hua Ching. *Tao, The Subtle Universal Law and Integral Way of Life.* Santa Monica, California: SevenStar Communications, 1985.

*Ni, Maoshing. *Chinese Herbology Made Easy.* Santa Monica, California: SevenStar Communications, 1986.

*Pang, T.Y. *Chinese Herbal: An Introduction.* East Sound, Washington: T'ai Chi School of Philosophy and Art, 1982.

*Reid, Daniel P. *Chinese Herbal Medicine.* Boston, Massachusetts: Shambhala, 1987.

*Teeguarden, Ron. *Chinese Tonic Herbs.* New York: Japan Publications, 1985.

*Tierra, Lesley. *The Herbs of Life: Health and Healing Using Western and Chinese Techniques.* Freedom, California: The Crossing Press, 1992. (*This book is a treasure!*)

*Tierra, Michael. *The Way of Herbs*. New York: Washington Square Press, 1980.

*Tierra, Michael. *Planetary Herbology*. Santa Fe, New Mexico: Lotus Press, 1988.

*Unschuld, Paul U. *Medicine in China: History of Pharmaceutics*. Berkeley, California: University of California Press, 1986.

*Zhang Enqin.. *Chinese Medicated Diet*. Shanghai, China: Publishing House of Shanghai College of Traditional Chinese Medicine, 1988.

Two companion cookbooks to *The Tao of Nutrition* that utilize the principles of Chinese Nutrition, and include recipes with Chinese *food herbs:*

*Chuang, Lily. *Chinese Vegetarian Delights: Sugar and Dairy Free Cookbook*. Santa Monica, California: SevenStar Communications, 1987.

*Chuang, Lily and Cathy McNease. *101 Vegetarian Delights*. Santa Monica, California: SevenStar Communications, 1992.

For additional healthy recipes, we suggest the following cookbooks:

Colbin, Annemarie. *The Book of Whole Meals*. New York: Ballantine Books, 1983.

Estella, Mary. *Natural Foods Cookbook: Vegetarian Dairy-Free Cuisine*. New York: Japan Publications, 1985.

Fessler, Stella Lau. *Chinese Meatless Cooking*. New York: Signet Books, 1983.

Hagler, Louise. *Tofu Cookery*. Summertown, Tennessee: The Book Publishing Co., 1982.

Hoshijo, Kathy. *Kathy Cooks Naturally.* San Francisco: Harbor Publishing Co., 1981.

Jacobs, Barbara and Leonard. *Cooking with Seitan.* New York: Japan Publications, 1986.

Lappe, Frances Moore. *Diet for a Small Planet.* New York: Ballantine Books, 1971.

Lin, Florence. *Florence Lin's Chinese Vegetarian Cookbook.* Boulder, Colorado: Shambhala, 1983.

Pickarski, Brother Ron. *Friendly Foods.* Berkeley, California: Ten Speed Press, 1991

Robertson, Laurel, Carol Flinders, and Bronwen Godfrey. *Laurel's Kitchen.* Berkeley, California: Nilgiri Press, 1976.

Saltzman, Joanne. *Amazing Grains: Creating Vegetarian Main Dishes from Whole Grains.* Tiburon, California: H.J.Kramer, 1990.

Shurtleff, William and Akiko Aoyagi. *The Book of Tofu.* Brookline, Massachusetts: Autumn Press, 1975.

Weber, Marcea. *Whole Meals.* Newberry Park, California: Prism Press, 1983.

CHINESE FOOD/HERB SOURCES

Some of the foods and herbs mentioned are only available from an Oriental market, health food store or specialty food store. Chinatown in any large city is sure to have the foods mentioned. The following stores are sources for Chinese herbs and foods mentioned in this text:

Best Blends Herb Company P.O.Box 1329, Ojai, Ca. 93023 (805)646-4466 (MAIL ORDER)

Great China Herb Company, 857 Washington St., San Francisco, Ca. 94108, (415) 982-2195

Herb King Chinese Herb Center, 3010 Lincoln Blvd. Santa Monica, Ca. 90405, (310)399-4470

Hong Kong Supermarket, 127 N. Garfield St., Monterey Park, Ca. 91754, (818)280-0520

Kowloon Market, 750 N. Hill St., Los Angeles, Ca. 90012, (213)488-0264

Ranch Market, 988 N. Hill St., Los Angeles, Ca. 90012, (213)625-3399

Ranch Market, 140 Valley Blvd., San Gabriel, Ca. 91776, (818)307-8899

Man Wah Supermarket, 9673 Bolsa Ave., Westminster, Ca. 92683, (714)531-4666

Mayee Ginseng Company, 943 N.Hill St., Los Angeles, Ca. 90012, (213) 687-3269

T. S. Emporium (Tak Shing Hong), 821 No. Broadway, Los Angeles, Ca. 90012, (213)680-1887

Wing Fung Tai Ginseng Company, 811 N. Broadway, Los Angeles, Ca. 90012, (213) 617-0699

General Index

A

A.I.D.S. 16, 118, 127

abdominal distention 51, 53, 78, 74, 97, 105

abdominal pain 38, 41, 65, 102, 105 - 106, 108 - 109, 135, 140, 171

abscess 39, 41, 46, 49 - 50, 53, 55, 60, 89, 95 - 96, 110 - 111

acid 29, 52 - 53, 75, 107, 168

acne 80, 117 - 118

acupuncture 9, 17, 20, 121, 163

alcohol (see also wine) 28, 36 - 37, 48, 52, 59, 64, 68, 70 - 72, 74, 113, 118 - 119, 122 - 123, 127, 129, 131 - 132, 138 - 139, 145 - 146, 148 - 149, 153, 157 - 158, 161 - 164, 166 - 167, 169, 171

alfalfa sprout 27, 117, 135, 138, 212

allergy 44 - 45, 83, 100, 113, 120, 123, 171

almond 24, 57, 85, 109, 124, 215

aloe vera 33, 37, 48, 80, 82, 117 - 119

American Ginseng 136 - 137, 214

anemia 28, 61, 63, 68, 70, 81, 94, 98, 100, 103

anger 7, 10, 17, 210

anise 2, 102, 126, 164, 215

anorexia 29, 80, 120 - 121, 148

anti-bacterial (also see bacteria) 49, 89

anti-viral (see also virus) 39, 49

antidote to drugs 48, 108

appendicitis 54, 95

appetite 7, 23, 29, 35, 42, 44, 60, 64 - 65, 68, 73 - 74, 78, 87, 89, 93, 99, 106, 120, 126, 154, 161, 171

apple 58, 70, 72, 111, 130 - 131, 134 - 136, 139 - 141, 143, 148, 151 - 152, 155, 157, 167, 212

apricot 15, 31, 57 - 59, 92, 119, 124 - 125, 129 - 130, 132 - 133, 135, 212

apricot kernels 15, 57, 59, 119, 124, 129 - 130, 132 - 133

arteriosclerosis 27, 113, 207

arthritis 47, 49 - 51, 54, 63 - 64, 92, 95, 97, 108, 110, 113 - 114, 121 - 123

ascites 53, 57, 143, 207

Asian pear (see also pear-apple) 70 - 71, 212

asparagus 27, 29, 126, 136, 212

asthma 42 - 43, 59, 63, 85 - 86, 92, 95, 123 - 124, 208, 211

astringent 13 - 15, 66, 71, 88, 110, 207

azuki bean (see also red bean) 40, 126, 131 - 132, 142 - 143, 148, 161, 163 - 164, 169, 215

B

back pain 40, 54, 68, 86, 95, 99, 102, 106, 127, 154, 156 - 157, 166

bacteria 8, 17, 19, 38, 49, 89, 110, 139, 157, 209, 211

baldness 55, 108

bamboo shaving 159, 214

epilepsy 36

essence 9, 11, 73, 156

exercise 17 - 18, 20 - 21, 107, 128,
131, 138, 146, 148, 153, 163,
169, 207, 210

eye hemorrhage 75, 113

eye weakness 32

eyes 10, 13, 30 - 32, 36, 46, 73, 75,
85, 112, 128, 144, 210

F

facial mask 80

fasting 19

fear 11, 17, 210

fennel 2, 40, 63, 75, 80, 107, 140,
154 - 155, 163, 215

ferocious appetite 7, 93

fetal retention 82

fever 48 - 49, 57, 66, 88, 98, 110,
124, 128, 133 - 134, 148, 157,
160 - 161, 167, 207 - 211

fibroid tumor 50

fig 63, 124 - 126, 131 - 132, 135 -
136, 139 - 140, 147, 155, 164,
170, 212

filbert 87, 215

fish 2, 24, 55, 62, 69, 97, 99, 111,
118 - 120, 122, 125 - 126, 129 -
130, 132, 134 - 137, 141, 143 -
144, 147, 149 - 153, 156, 164,
171 - 172, 215

fish bone 62, 111

Five Elements 12, 216 - 218

flu 63 - 64, 78, 211

fluid in the abdomen (see also
ascites) 76

food poisoning (see also seafood
poisoning) 57, 89, 103 - 104,
108, 112, 140

Food Pyramid 24

food retention 28 - 30, 37, 46, 51,
54, 74 - 75, 82, 102, 112

frequent urination 73, 81, 86 - 88,
95, 156

frostbite 29, 31, 38, 64

fruits 21 - 22, 24, 58, 120, 123, 125
- 127, 139 - 140, 153, 156, 212
- 213

G

gall bladder 35, 79, 168

gallstones 35, 77, 168

Ganoderma mushroom 42, 118, 213

garlic 7, 14, 39, 94, 99, 111, 118,
120 - 122, 126 - 128, 131 - 134,
137, 139 - 141, 143 - 145, 148,
151 - 152, 161 - 162, 165, 171 -
172, 213

gas 13, 41, 53, 64, 81, 87, 102, 106,
207, 209

gastritis 41, 209

ginger 2, 7, 14, 28, 34 - 35, 37 - 39,
43, 45, 47, 50, 54, 64, 75, 78,
81, 92, 94, 99 - 100, 103 - 105,
108 - 109, 111, 119 - 122, 126,
129 - 134, 137, 139 - 141, 143,
145, 149 - 150, 154, 156, 159 -
160, 162 - 163, 166, 170 - 171,
215

glaucoma 144

goiter 15, 50, 54 - 55, 60

goldenseal root 38, 214

Resources for Your Healthy Life

BOOKS

101 Vegetarian Delights - by Lily Chuang and Cathy McNease - A lovely cookbook with recipes as tasty as they are healthy. Features multi-cultural recipes, appendices on Chinese herbs and edible flowers and a glossary of special foods. Over 40 illustrations. B101v 0-937064-13-0 PAPERBACK 176P $12.95

The Yellow Emperor's Classic of Medicine - *NEW!* - by Maoshing Ni, Ph.D. The *Neijing* is one of the most important classics of Taoism, as well as the highest authority on traditional Chinese medicine. Written in the form of a discourse between Yellow Emperor and his ministers, this book contains a wealth of knowledge on holistic medicine and how human life can attune itself to receive natural support. BYELLO 1-57062-080-6 PAPERBACK 316P $16.00

The Eight Treasures: Energy Enhancement Exercise - *NEW!* -by Maoshing Ni, Ph. D. The Eight Treasures is an ancient system of energy enhancing movements based on the natural motion of the universe. It can be practiced by anyone at any fitness level, is non-impact, simple to do, and appropriate for all ages. It is recommended that this book be used with its companion videotape. BEIGH 0-937064-55-6 Paperback 208p $17.95

Power of Natural Healing - This book is for anyone wanting to heal themselves or others. Methods include revitalization with acupuncture and herbs, *Tai Chi, Chi Kung (Chi Gong)*, sound, color, movement, visualization and meditation. BHEAL 0-937064-31-9 PAPERBACK 230P $14.95

Strength From Movement: Mastering Chi - by Hua-Ching Ni, Daoshing Ni and Maoshing Ni. - *Chi*, the vital power of life, can be developed and cultivated within yourself to help support your healthy, happy life. This book gives the deep reality of different useful forms of *chi* exercise and which types are best for certain types of people. Includes samples of several popular exercises. BSTRE 0-937064-73-4 PAPERBACK WITH 42 PHOTOGRAPHS 256P $16.95.

Attune Your Body with *Dao-In* - The ancient Taoist predecessor to *Tai Chi Chuan*, these movements can be performed sitting and lying down to guide and refine your energy. Includes meditations and massage for a complete integral fitness program. To be used in conjunction with the video. BDAOI 0-937065-40-8 PAPERBACK WITH PHOTOGRAPHS 144P $14.95

The Tao of Nutrition - by Maoshing Ni, Ph.D., with Cathy McNease, B.S., M.H. - Learn how to take control of your health with good eating. Over 100 common foods are discussed with their energetic properties and therapeutic functions listed. Food remedies for numerous common ailments are also presented. BNUTR 0-937064-66-1 PAPERBACK 214P $14.50

Chinese Vegetarian Delights - by Lily Chuang - An extraordinary collection of recipes based on principles of traditional Chinese nutrition. Meat, sugar, dairy products and fried foods are excluded. BCHIV 0-937064-13-0 PAPERBACK 104P $7.50

Chinese Herbology Made Easy - by Maoshing Ni, Ph.D. - This text provides an overview of Oriental medical theory, in-depth descriptions of each herb category, over 300 black and white photographs, extensive tables of individual herbs for easy reference and an index of pharmaceutical names. BCHIH 0-937064-12-2 PAPERBACK 202P $14.50

Crane Style Chi Gong Book - By Daoshing Ni, Ph.D. - Standing meditative exercises practiced for healing. Combines breathing techniques, movement, and mental imagery to guide the smooth flow of energy. To be used with or without the videotape. BCRAN 0-937064-10-6 SPIRAL-BOUND 55P $10.95

VIDEOTAPES

Self-Healing *Chi Gong* (VHS Video) - Strengthen your own self-healing powers. These effective mind-body exercises strengthen and balance each of your five major organ systems. Two hours of practical demonstrations and information lectures. VSHCG VHS VIDEO 120 MINUTES $39.95

Taoist Eight Treasures (VHS) - By Maoshing Ni, Ph.D. - Unique to the Ni family, these 32 exercises open and refine the energy flow and strengthen one's vitality. Combines stretching, toning and energy conducting with deep breathing Book also available. VEIGH VHS VIDEO 105 MINUTES $39.95

***T'ai Chi Ch'uan* I & II (VHS)** - By Maoshing Ni, Ph.D. - This style, called the style of Harmony, is a distillation of the Yang, Chen and Wu styles. It integrates physical movement with internal energy and helps promote longevity and self-cultivation. VTAI1 VHS VIDEO PART 1 60 MINUTES $39.95 • VTAI2 VHS VIDEO PART 2 60 MINUTES $39.95

Attune Your Body with *Dao-In* (VHS) - by Master Hua-Ching Ni. - The ancient Taoist predecessor to *Tai Chi Chuan*. Performed sitting and lying down, these moves unblock, guide and refine energy. Includes meditations and massage for a complete integral fitness program. VDAOI VHS VIDEO 60 MINUTES $39.95

***T'ai Chi Ch'uan*: An Appreciation (VHS)** - by Hua-Ching Ni. - "Gentle Path," "Sky Journey" and "Infinite Expansion" are three esoteric styles handed down by highly achieved masters and are shown in an uninterrupted format. Not an instructional video. VAPPR VHS VIDEO 30 MINUTES $24.95

Crane Style *Chi Gong* (VHS) - by Dr. Daoshing Ni, Ph.D. - These ancient exercises are practiced for healing purposes. They integrate movement, mental imagery and breathing techniques. To be used with the book. VCRAN VHS VIDEO 120 MINUTES $39.95

Natural Living and the Universal Way (VHS) – Interview of Hua-Ching Ni in the show "Asian-American Focus" hosted by Lily Chu. Dialogue on common issues of everyday life and practical wisdom. VINTE VHS VIDEO 30 MINUTES $15.95

Movement Arts for Emotional Health (VHS) - Interview of Hua-Ching Ni in the show "Asian-American Focus" hosted by Lily Chu. Dialogue on emotional health and energy exercise that are fundamental to health and well-being. VMOVE VHS VIDEO 30 MINUTES $15.95

AUDIO CASSETTES

Invocations for Health, Longevity and Healing a Broken Heart - By Maoshing Ni, Ph.D. - "Thinking is louder than thunder." This cassette guides you through a series of invocations to channel and conduct your own healing energy and vital force. AINVO AUDIO 30 MINUTES $9.95

Stress Release with Chi Gong - By Maoshing Ni, Ph.D. - This audio cassette guides you through simple breathing techniques that enable you to release stress and tension that are a common cause of illness today. ACHIS AUDIO 30 MINUTES $9.95

Pain Management with Chi Gong - By Maoshing Ni, Ph.D. - Using visualization and deep-breathing techniques, this cassette offers methods for overcoming pain by invigorating your energy flow and unblocking obstructions that cause pain. ACHIP AUDIO 30 MINUTES $9.95

Tao Teh Ching Cassette Tapes - The classic work of Lao Tzu in this two-cassette set is a companion to the book translated by Hua-Ching Ni. Professionally recorded and read by Robert Rudelson. ATAOT 120 MINUTES $12.95

Teachings of the Universal Way
by Hua-Ching Ni

NEW BOOKS

Spring Thunder: Awaken the Hibernating Power of Life - Humans need to be periodically awakened from a spiritual hibernation in which the awareness of life's reality is deeply forgotten. To awaken your deep inner life, this book offers the practice of Natural Meditation, the enlightening teachings of Yen Shi, and Master Ni's New Year Message. BSPRI 0-937064-77-7 PAPERBACK, 168 P $12.95

The Universal Path of Natural Life - The way to make your life enduring is to harmonize with the nature of the universe. By doing so, you expand beyond your limits to reach universal life. This book is the third in the series called *The Course for Total Health*. BUNIV 0-937064-76-9 PAPERBACK, 104P $9.50

Power of Positive Living How do you know if your spirit is healthy? You do not need to be around sickness to learn what health is. When you put aside the cultural and social confusion around you, you can rediscover your true self and restore your natural health. This is the second book of *The Course for Total Health*. BPOWE 0-937064-90-4 PAPERBACK 80P $8.50

The Gate to Infinity - People who have learned spiritually through years without real progress will be thoroughly guided by the important discourse in this book. Master Ni also explains Natural Meditation. Editors recommend that all serious spiritual students who wish to increase their spiritual potency read this one. BGATE 0-937064-68-8 PAPERBACK 208P $13.95

Self-Reliance and Constructive Change - Natural spiritual reality is independent of concept. Thus dependence upon religious convention, cultural notions and political ideals must be given up to reach full spiritual potential. The Declaration of Spiritual Independence affirms spiritual self-authority and true wisdom as the highest attainments of life. This is the first book in *The Course for Total Health*. BSELF 0-937064-85-8 PAPERBACK 64P $7.00

Concourse of All Spiritual Paths - All religions, in spite of their surface difference, in their essence return to the great oneness. Hua-Ching Ni looks at what traditional religions offer us today and suggests how to go beyond differences to discover the depth of universal truth. BCONC 0-937064-61-0 PAPERBACK 184P $15.95.

OTHER PUBLICATIONS: PRACTICAL LIVING

Harmony - The Art of Life - The emphasis in this book is on creating harmony within ourselves so that we can find it in relationships with other people and with our environment. BHARM 0-937064-37-8 PAPERBACK 208P $14.95

Moonlight in the Dark Night - This book contains wisdom on how to control emotions, including how to manage love relationships so that they do not impede one's spiritual achievement. BMOON 0-937064-44-0 PAPERBACK 168P $12.95

The Key to Good Fortune: Refining Your Spirit - $12.95

Ageless Counsel for Modern Life - $15.95.

8,000 Years of Wisdom, Volume I - $18.50 • **Volume II:** $12.50

The Time is Now for a Better Life and a Better World - P $10.95

Spiritual Messages from a Buffalo Rider, A Man of Tao - $12.95

Golden Message - by Daoshing and Maoshing Ni - $11.95

SPIRITUAL DEVELOPMENT

The Mystical Universal Mother - Hua-Ching Ni responds to the questions of his female students through the example of his mother and other historical and mythical women. He focuses on the feminine aspect of both sexes and on the natural relationship between men and women. BMYST 0-937064-45-9 PAPERBACK 240P $14.95

Eternal Light - Dedicated to Yo San Ni, a renowned healer and teacher, and father of Hua-Ching Ni. An intimate look at the lifestyle of a spiritually centered family. BETER 0-937064-38-6 PAPERBACK 208P $14.95

Life and Teaching of Two Immortals, Volume 1: Kou Hong - $12.95.

Life and Teaching of Two Immortals, Volume 2: Chen Tuan - $12.95

The Way, the Truth and the Light -PAPERBACK $14.95 • HARDCOVER 232P $22.95

Quest of Soul - $11.95

Nurture Your Spirits - $12.95

Internal Alchemy: The Natural Way to Immortality - $15.95

Mysticism: Empowering the Spirit Within - $13.95

Internal Growth through Tao - $13.95

Essence of Universal Spirituality - $19.95

Guide to Inner Light -$12.95

Stepping Stones for Spiritual Success - $12.95.

The Story of Two Kingdoms - $14.50

The Gentle Path of Spiritual Progress - $12.95.

Footsteps of the Mystical Child - $9.50

TIMELESS CLASSICS

The Complete Works of Lao Tzu - The *Tao Teh Ching* is one of the most widely translated and cherished works of literature. Its timeless wisdom provides a bridge to the subtle spiritual truth and aids harmonious and peaceful living. Plus the only authentic written translation of the *Hua Hu Ching*, a later work of Lao Tzu which was lost to the general public for a thousand years. BCOMP 0-937064-00-9 PAPERBACK 212P $13.95

The Book of Changes and the Unchanging Truth - Revised Edition - This version of the timeless classic *I Ching* is heralded as the standard for modern times. A unique presentation including profound illustrative commentary and details of the book's underlying natural science and philosophy from a world-renowned expert. BBOOK 0-937064-81-5 HARDCOVER 669P $35.00

Workbook for Spiritual Development - $14.95

The Esoteric Tao Teh Ching - $13.95

The Way of Integral Life -PAPERBACK $14.00 • HARDCOVER $20.00.

Enlightenment: Mother of Spiritual Independence - PAPERBACK $12.50 • HARDCOVER $22.00.

Attaining Unlimited Life - PAPERBACK $18.00; $25.00

The Taoist Inner View of the Universe - $14.95

Tao, the Subtle Universal Law - $12.95

MUSIC AND MISCELLANEOUS

Colored Dust - Sung by Gaille. Poetry by Hua-Ching Ni. - CASSETTE $10.98, ADUST2 COMPACT DISC $15.95

Poster of Master Lu - $10.95

POCKET BOOKLETS

Guide to Your Total Well-Being - Simple useful practices for self-development, aid for your spiritual growth and guidance for all aspects of life. Exercise, food, sex, emotional balancing, meditation. BWELL 0-937064-78-5 PAPERBACK 48P $4.00

Progress Along the Way: Life, Service and Realization - The guiding power of human life is the association between the developed mind and the achieved soul which contains love, rationality, conscience and everlasting value. BPROG 0-937-064-79-3 PAPERBACK 64P $4.00

The Light of All Stars Illuminates the Way - Through generations of searching, various achieved ones found the best application of the Way in their lives. This booklet contains their discovery. BSTAR 0-937064-80-7 48P $4.00

Less Stress, More Happiness - Helpful information for identifying and relieving stress in your life including useful techniques such as invocations, breathing and relaxation, meditation, exercise, nutrition and lifestyle balancing. BLESS 0-937064-55-06 48P $3.00

Integral Nutrition - Nutrition is an integral part of a healthy, natural life. Includes information on how to assess your basic body type, food preparation, energetic properties of food, nutrition and digestion. BNUTR 0-937064-84-X 32P $3.00

The Heavenly Way - Straighten Your Way (*Tai Shan Kan Yin Pien*) and The Silent Way of Blessing (*Yin Chia Wen*) are the main sources of inspiration for this booklet that sets the cornerstone for a mature, healthy life. BHEAV 0-937064-03-3 PAPERBACK 42P $2.50

SevenStar Mail Order Form

Name: _____

Address: _____

City: _____ State: _____ Zip: _____

Phone (daytime): _____ (Evening): _____

Qty.	Stock #	Title	Price ea.	Subtotal

Sales tax (CA residents only): _____

Shipping: _____

Total: _____

Payment: Check, money order or credit card

Card number: _____
                                                  Exp. date

Signature: _____

Shipping: via UPS in the continental United States. $5.50 for first item and 50¢ for each additional item. The *I Ching* counts as 3 items. Please call for international shipping rates to all other locations.

Telephone orders, questions or catalog requests: 800/578-9526
Website: www.taostar.com   E-mail: taostar@taostar.com

Mail form with payment (US funds only) to:
13315 W. Washington Blvd. Suite 200 • Los Angeles, California 90066

Spiritual Study and Teaching Through the College of Tao

The College of Tao and SevenStar Communications were formally established in California in the 1970's, yet this tradition is a very old spiritual culture containing centuries of human spiritual growth. Its central goal is to offer healthy spiritual education to all people. This time-tested school values the spiritual development of each individual self and passes down its guidance and experience.

The College of Tao is a school which has no walls. The big human society is its classroom. Your own teaching and service is the class you attend; thus students grow from their lives and from studying the guidance of the Integral Way. The goal of the school is to help individuals develop themselves and become Mentors of the Integral Way. A Mentor is any individual who is spiritually self-responsible and who sets up the model of a healthy and complete life for oneself and others.

Any interested individual is welcome to join and learn to grow for oneself. The Correspondence Course/Self-Study Program can be useful to you. The Program, which is based on Master Ni's books and videotapes, gives people who wish to study on their own or are too far from a center or volunteer teachers an opportunity to study the learning of the Way at their own speed. The outline of how to participate in the Correspondence Course/Self-Study Program can be found at the end of the book, *The Golden Message*.

It is recommended that all Mentors of the Integral Way use the self-study program in *The Golden Message* to educate themselves. They can teach special skills which are certified by the College of Tao. Those who engage in teaching with Master Ni's materials must follow the Mentor Service Regulations of the College of Tao. To receive recognition from the College of Tao for teaching activity, a Mentor must register with the College.

If you are interested in the Universal Society of the Integral Way Correspondence Course/Self-Study Program, write: College of Tao • PO Box 1222 • El Prado, NM 87529

Mail to: USIW • 13315 W. Washington Blvd. Suite 200 • Los Angeles, CA 90066

____ I wish to be put on the mailing list of the USIW to be notified of educational activities.

____ I wish to receive a list of registered Mentors teaching in my area or country.

____ I am interested in joining/forming a study group in my area.

____ I am interested in becoming a Mentor of the USIW.

Name _____

Address _____

City _____ State _____ Zip _____

Herbs Used by Ancient Masters

The pursuit of everlasting youth or immortality throughout human history is an innate human desire. Long ago, Chinese esoteric Taoists went to the high mountains to contemplate nature, strengthen their bodies, empower their minds and develop their spirit. From their studies and cultivation, they China alchemy and chemistry, herbology and acupuncture, the I Ching, astrology, martial arts and T'ai Chi Ch'uan, Chi Gong and many other useful kinds of knowledge.

Most important, they handed down in secrecy methods for attaining longevity and spiritual immortality. There were different levels of approach; one was to use a collection of food herb formulas that were only available to highly achieved Taoist masters. They used these food herbs to increase energy and heighten vitality. This treasured collection of herbal formulas remained within the Ni family for centuries.

Now, through Traditions of Tao, the Ni family makes these foods available for you to use to assist the foundation of your own positive development. It is only with a strong foundation that expected results are produced from diligent cultivation. For further information about Traditions of Tao herbal products, please call or mail this form to:

Traditions of Tao
13315 W. Washington Boulevard Suite 200
Los Angeles, CA 90066
(800) 772-0222

Please send me a Traditions of Tao brochure.

Name_____

Address _____

City _____ State _____ Zip _____

Phone (day) _____ (evening) _____

Yo San University of Traditional Chinese Medicine

"Not just a medical career, but a life-time commitment to raising one's spiritual standard."

Thank you for your support and interest in our publications and services. It is by your patronage that we continue to offer you the practical knowledge and wisdom from this venerable Taoist tradition.

Because of your sustained interest in Taoism, in January 1989 we formed Yo San University of Traditional Chinese Medicine, a non-profit educational institution under the direction of founder Master Ni, Hua-Ching. Yo San University is the continuation of 38 generations of Ni family practitioners who handed down knowledge and wisdom from father to son. Its purpose is to train and graduate practitioners of the highest caliber in Traditional Chinese Medicine, which includes acupuncture, herbology and spiritual development.

We view Traditional Chinese Medicine as the application of spiritual development. Its foundation is the spiritual capability to know life, to diagnose a person's problem and how to cure it. We teach students how to care for themselves and others, emphasizing the integration of traditional knowledge and modern science. Yo San University offers a complete Master's degree program approved by the California State Department of Education that provides an excellent education in Traditional Chinese Medicine and meets all requirements for state licenser.

We invite you to inquire into our university for a creative and rewarding career as a holistic physician. Classes are also open to persons interested only in self-enrichment. For more information, please fill out the form below and send it to:

Yo San University
of Traditional Chinese Medicine
13315 W. Washington Boulevard Suite 200
Los Angeles, CA 90066

❑ Please send me information on the Masters degree program in Traditional Chinese Medicine.

❑ Please send me information on health workshops and seminars.

❑ Please send me information on continuing education for acupuncturists and health professionals.

Name_____

Address _____

City _____ State _____ Zip _____

Phone (day) _____ (evening) _____